# Handbook of Evidence-based Veterinary Medicine

Peter D. Cockcroft MA VetMB MSc DCHP DVM&S MRCVS
Mark A. Holmes PhD, MA, VetMB, MRCVS
*Epidemiology and Informatics Unit*
*Department of Clinical Veterinary Medicine*
*University of Cambridge*

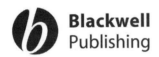

**Blackwell**
Publishing

© 2003 by Blackwell Publishing Ltd
Editorial Offices:
9600 Garsington Road, Oxford OX4 2DQ, UK
  Tel: +44 (0)1865 776868
108 Cowley Road, Oxford OX4 1JF, UK
  Tel: +44 (0)1865 791100
Blackwell Publishing Inc., 350 Main Street, Malden,
MA 02148-5018, USA
  Tel: +1 781 388 8250
Iowa State Press, a Blackwell Publishing Company,
2121 State Avenue, Ames, Iowa 50014-8300, USA
  Tel: +1 515 292 0140
Blackwell Munksgaard, 1 Rosenørns Allé, P.O. Box
227, DK-1502 Copenhagen V, Denmark
  Tel: +45 77 33 33 33
Blackwell Publishing Asia Pty Ltd, 550 Swanston
Street, Carlton South, Victoria 3053, Australia
  Tel: +61 (0)3 9347 0300
Blackwell Verlag, Kurfürstendamm 57, 10707 Berlin,
Germany
  Tel: +49 (0)30 32 79 060
Blackwell Publishing, 10 rue Casimir Delavigne,
75006 Paris, France
  Tel: +33 1 53 10 33 10

First published 2003

A catalogue record for this title is available
from the British Library

ISBN 1-4051-0890-8

Library of Congress
Cataloging-in-Publication Data
is available

Set in 10/12pt Optima
By DP Photosetting, Alyesbury, Bucks
Printed and bound in Great Britain by
TJ International, Padstow, Cornwall

For further information on
Blackwell Publishing, visit our website:
www.blackwellpublishing.com

## DEDICATION

For Elizabeth, Edward and Simon (PDC)

For John and Pandora, my parents without whom I wouldn't have been able to write this book, and for Henry, my son, who made it worth writing (MAH)

# CONTENTS

# PREFACE

Evidence-based medicine has been defined as 'the conscientious, explicit and judicious use of current best evidence in making decisions about the individual patients'. This means integrating individual clinical expertise with the best available clinical evidence from systematic research (Sackett *et al.* 2000). In veterinary medicine a broader, simpler definition may be appropriate, 'Evidence-based veterinary medicine is the use of current best evidence in making clinical decisions'.

This book is for veterinary surgeons at any stage of their training or career who want to learn about evidence-based veterinary medicine (EBVM), but it has been written particularly for non-academic practitioners. It is an attempt to help veterinary surgeons practise EBVM and improve the quality of care for animal patients and provide informed choices for owners. This may take the form of knowing the specificity and sensitivity of a diagnostic test, understanding your own clinical reasoning, interpreting a diagnostic decision support system or understanding what an article about therapy/harm/prognosis is telling you. The practice of EBVM should form part of lifelong, self-directed learning without which you may rapidly become dangerously out of date.

EBVM may be described as 'Just in time learning' (as opposed to 'Just in case learning'), 'Science into practice' or 'From publication to patient'. Whatever jargon is used, it is now time to accept that there is a range of skills that are required to apply best practice to our patients that we may not have. These skills include computer skills, a knowledge of experimental design, the ability to ask questions and transform information needs into questions to which the answer may be found in the literature, and an ability to understand and critically appraise the evidence being presented. We need to have an EBVM toolkit in our armoury of professional skills.

This book aims to explain what EBVM is, and how it can be applied to veterinary practice.

By reading this book you should achieve the following objectives:

- Know how to transform information needs into a series of clinical questions that can be answered
- Know how to search for best available external evidence
- Know how to critically appraise the evidence for its validity and importance
- Know how to apply it in clinical practice
- Understand the process of diagnosis and clinical diagnostic decision support systems.

The authors hope you find the book both useful and interesting.

Peter D. Cockcroft
Mark A. Holmes

## Reference

Sackett, D.L., Straus, S.E., Richardson, S.W. and Rosenberg, W. (2000) *Evidence-Based Medicine: How to Practice and Teach EBM.* Churchill Livingstone, Edinburgh.

## Acknowledgements

The authors would like to thank Antonia Seymour and Lindsie Court of Blackwell Publishing for their guidance and support and Dr Cerian Webb for her advice on modelling in chapter 9. Mark Holmes would also like to thank the Leverhulme Trust for his Leverhulme Study Abroad Fellowship during which the book was written.

# INTRODUCTION

'Progress in the field of evidence-based veterinary medicine (EBVM) will become a bench mark of our professional progress in the twenty-first century' (Keene 2000)

## 1.1   Who is this book for?

This book has been written for veterinary surgeons in non-academic, non-referral practices. A typical veterinary surgeon in such a practice is highly competent, but has to work hard to balance the needs of their business, their family, and their vocation. Our typical veterinary surgeon undertakes formal continuing professional development (CPD) in the form of attendance at courses, meetings and conferences. They purchase the latest editions of textbooks and subscribe to several journals. Although they have little time for reading they try to keep up to date by consulting their books and course notes when faced with unusual cases, and they read articles from the journals. The articles they read are mainly review articles with titles that often include phrases such as 'advances in', 'updates on', 'new techniques in', and 'a new approach to'. These veterinary surgeons know that there is a massive base of scientific work that underpins the work that they do and they rely on the 'experts' who write the books, lecture at meetings, and teach on courses to analyse and appraise this body of scientific work before it is passed into the realm of current best practice.

The benefits that will accrue from the implementation of EBVM include improvements in their levels of knowledge, the focus of that knowledge, and greater satisfaction in their practice of veterinary medicine. Instead of routinely reviewing the contents of dozens of journals for interesting articles, EBVM suggests you target your reading to issues related to specific patient problems. EBVM converts the abstract exercise of reading and appraising the literature into the pragmatic process of using the literature to benefit individual patients while simultaneously expanding the clinician's knowledge base. Developing clinical questions and then searching current databases may be a more productive way of keeping your knowledge base current and appropriate to your patients' needs.

## 1.2   Who isn't this book for?

This book is not really intended for the academics and specialists who, knowing a little about it already, may regard EBVM with a weary resignation. It is unlikely that their adoption of EBVM would affect the way they practise. They would, quite rightly, claim to have practised EBVM before it became a trendy repackaging of clinical epidemiology. They will be practising to a very high standard, armed with a detailed knowledge of the current literature in their field. They are luckier than more broadly-based practitioners because as specialists, they don't have quite so much literature to read, and with their higher background knowledge they find it easier to understand and apply it to their work. At a subliminal level they might feel a little threatened by it. They may just dismiss the notion that general veterinary practitioners will ever have the time, skills or inclination to use the primary scientific literature. They may also point out that while the medical profession can call upon a mass of scientific literature covering every clinical situation, the veterinary literature is patchy in its coverage of even common diseases.

Although this book is not intended for the academics and specialists, the authors hope that they will recognise both the feasibility of the practice of EBVM and the advantages to be gained from it in non-academic practice.

## 1.3   What do we mean by EBVM? A brief description

The widely quoted definition of evidence-based medicine is that 'Evidence-based medicine is the conscientious, explicit and judicious use of current best evidence in making decisions about the care of individual patients'. This means integrating individual clinical expertise and the best available external clinical evidence from systematic research (Sackett *et al.* 2000).

This succinct, and some would say obvious, definition of what we all try to do anyway, belies the more profound philosophy behind EBVM. At its heart is the confidence in the scientific methodology that has developed over the centuries to enable us to distinguish what is likely to be true from what is likely to be false (or unproven). The evidence upon which we base our faith in our clinical decisions is derived from the scientific literature. Practitioners of EBVM develop the skills to find and appraise the literature pertinent to the cases we see, and apply this evidence to the clinical decisions we make.

If this was a book for human doctors we might stop there, but as veterinary surgeons we will frequently find ourselves in situations where there is no primary scientific evidence on which to base our decisions. We will have evidence in the form of expert opinion, case reports, personal experience and other non-literature based sources which should also be collated, assessed, and ranked in order to arrive at a decision.

The most important word in the definition of EBM is probably the word 'explicit'. When a practitioner of EBVM is asked how they chose one clinical option over another, they will be able to explain how and why the decision was made, having pursued an explicit and methodical process.

Finally, in this brief description, it should be said that EBVM is not about pursuing dogma. EBVM is not a home for evangelising zealots. EBVM is another facet of the constantly changing face of veterinary medicine. In general practice no two situations are ever identical, we are constantly forced to compromise, and juggle competing needs. At the end of each day, we examine our consciences to assess our performance. EBVM provides one yardstick for us to measure up to, whoever we believe we are accountable to.

## 1.4   Comparison of the traditional methods and EBVM

Rapid advances in knowledge constantly challenge our ability to provide the best and most current clinical information for patients. When faced by uncertainty as to the best and most current approach to a clinical problem we can choose from several options:

- We can rely on traditional tried and true protocols and resort to established habits to justify our decisions and give us confidence to proceed down a particular path and diagnosis. These may include: relying on our knowledge of pathophysiology, remembering unsystematic clinical observations of a previous case, tossing a coin to decide between two competing options, intelligent guesswork, doing nothing to avoid harm, remembering what you were taught 10 years ago (if you can), checking your dusty undergraduate notes, asking colleagues, referring to textbooks, browsing journals and doing a database search with an unstructured appraisal
- we can proceed on the basis of our personal experiences or clinical intuition
- we can seek the advice of an expert in the field
- we can rely on scientific EBVM.

The traditional approach suggests that:

- clinical experience is a valid way of gaining an understanding about diagnosis, prognosis and treatment
- pathophysiological rationale is a valid way of guiding treatments
- common sense and classical medical training are the only qualities needed to evaluate medical literature.

The EBVM approach suggests:

- personal experience may be misleading
- randomised studies are required to validate results because predictions based upon physiology may be wrong
- reading literature requires more than common sense to evaluate the evidence.

## 1.5   Why should we practise EBVM?

### 1.5.1   *Because we can*

One of the reasons that EBM has come of age is because of information technology. We no longer have to keep a card index of interesting papers and have access to veterinary school libraries in order to search the literature. With access to the Internet we can search through millions of papers in a matter of seconds. Having located a paper of interest we can often obtain a copy within a minute or two also via the Internet. Access is virtually free, and geographical distance is no issue. The future of our profession is in our new graduates who, almost without exception, now view the Internet as an everyday source of information, be it the programme at the local cinema, or the latest news from the State Veterinary Service.

Around 89% of veterinary practices in the UK are computerized. More than 50% of the practices have access to the Internet (Veterinary Marketing Association 2001). Vetstream is a commercially available information resource for veterinary surgeons. A survey of Vetstream users in 2001 (64 responders from 874 UK only subscribers (7.3%)) revealed that 82% of responding subscribers had access to the internet. The frequencies with which these subscribers used the internet were: rarely (23%), weekly (23%), once a day (29%) and several times a day (25%).

The use of Vetstream information programs by function in the last month prior to the survey is shown below. Selecting treatments and diagnosis were the functions most used.

| Function used in the last month | % |
| --- | --- |
| Selecting treatments | 81 |
| Diagnosing | 78 |
| Reviewing surgical techniques | 72 |
| Continuing professional development | 63 |
| Staff training | 46 |

### 1.5.2 *Because our clients can too*

Almost all the tools that enable us to locate the evidence we need are available to our clients too (and their lawyers). When we make clinical decisions that are questioned by clients following poor outcomes, we need to be able to account for our decisions. There will always be enormous scope, and need for clinical judgement, where possible backed up by the best scientific evidence. Effective communication of the evidence to clients helps them to make informed decisions and avoid unreal expectations.

### 1.5.3 *We need the information*

Information needed to solve a problem falls into three categories:

- information that is needed and is known
- information that is needed but is not known
- information needs that are not recognised.

With the volume of new information growing year on year, it is becoming impossible to keep up to date with all developments. It is unrealistic to expect veterinary surgeons to remember everything they need in order to practise since only the most commonly used information is readily available from memory. There is a need to identify information needs for a specific case and find the best evidence rather than try to retain a rudimentary knowledge. This need places the emphasis on how to look for information and evaluate it rather than trying to consume all the new developments, which is an impossible task. The growth in information is not simple addition to existing knowledge. Veterinary surgeons must identify and replace outdated and obsolete knowledge. Specialisation and information technology can assist this process but greater focus and selectivity in the knowledge we need to know is still required.

Decisions are made about diagnosis, prognosis, treatment and control of disease, and animal management. Veterinary surgeons use information to improve the accuracy of their decisions. Decision-making is based on their personal experience (internal experience) and other sources of experience (external experience), which may include the veterinary literature. The abilities to find the additional information and judge the quality of the information are essential skills (Radostits *et al.* 2000).

Usefulness of information sources commonly used by doctors is summarised in table 1.1 (Smith 1996).

A paper by Shaughnessy *et al.* (1994) put forward a formula for the usefulness of information:

$$\text{Usefulness of medical information} = \frac{\text{relevance} \times \text{validity}}{\text{work to access}}$$

- the relevance of any information is based on the frequency of your exposure to the problem and the type of evidence being presented
- the validity is the likelihood of the information being true
- the work to access the information is the time and effort that must be spent to extract and analyse for the strength of evidence it provides.

The ideal information source would be directly relevant, contain valid information, and be accessed with the minimum of effort.

A table of information sources for veterinary surgeons would not differ significantly from table 1.1. The central role of the veterinary surgeon is to meet the demands of patients, using the best knowledge accumulated over the last 5000 years. The information we hold in our memory may be out of date and wrong. Information sources vary depending on the type of information required. Patients' histories may be derived from owners, patient records, and laboratory data; disease prevalence data may come from local surveys or practice records; medical knowledge may come from textbooks, journals and electronic databases. A major challenge is to match the medical knowledge to the patient problem. In a survey of doctors, lack of time, cost, poor organisation, non-availability of sources, and a glut of sources of differing reliability were seen as barriers to finding information (Smith 1996). This survey found that:

**Table 1.1**    Sources of information used by human doctors.

| Information source | Relevance | Validity | Work to obtain information | Usefulness |
|---|---|---|---|---|
| *Future* | | | | |
| Evidence-based regularly updated electronic textbook | High | High | Low | High |
| Systematic journal review | High | High | Low | High |
| Portable summary of systematic reviews | High | High | Low | High |
| Internet online reviews | High | High | Low | High |
| *Now* | | | | |
| Drug reference book | High | Moderate | Low | High or moderate |
| Dedicated evidence-based journals | Moderate | High | Low | High or moderate |
| Colleagues | High | Moderate | Low | High or moderate |
| Standard textbook | High | Low | Low | Moderate |
| Standard journal review | High | Moderate | Low | Moderate |
| Collections of systematic reviews | Moderate but increasing | High | High but should fall | Moderate |
| Free medical newspapers | High | Low | Low | Moderate |
| Continuing medical education lectures | Moderate | Moderate | Low | Moderate |
| Continuing medical education small groups | High | Moderate | Moderate | Moderate |
| Consensus statements/reports | Moderate | Moderate | Low | Moderate |
| Clinical guidelines/protocols | Moderate | Moderate | Low | Moderate |
| Online searching | Moderate | High | High | Moderate |
| Journal articles | Low | High | High | Low |
| Drug advertising | Moderate | Low | Low | Low |
| Drug company representatives | High | Low | Low | Low |
| Mass media | Low | Low | Low | Low |
| Internet now | Low | Low | High | Low |

- information need arises regularly during consultations
- information need may go unrecognised
- most information needs go unanswered
- many questions arise about treatments and drugs

- clinicians are most likely to seek answers from other clinicians
- most of the questions generated can be answered from electronic sources but it is time consuming, costly and requires skill
- clinicians feel overwhelmed by the amount of information and find obtaining it and evaluating it difficult.

### 1.5.4   *Time for learning, a diminishing resource faced with expanding demands*

Traditional CPD involves attempting to predict what our future information needs are, finding a source for that information, and then filing away the information ready for when it is needed. For example, you may become aware that there are new antibiotics on the market, you see a review article in a journal, or an advertisement for an antimicrobial therapeutics meeting, you learn that some drugs you haven't used before might be useful for certain cases, you wait until you next get a suitable case, and then you apply the new knowledge. The EBVM approach is to look for the information in response to information needs for individual cases. The phrase 'Just in time knowledge' as opposed to 'Just in case knowledge' has been used to illustrate the new approach to these information needs. Everything that is learnt in this way is directly relevant to your practice, and the cases you see. Searching skills, and appraising skills have to be learnt, but once acquired you are maximising the efficiency of CPD time.

Within the human medical world there is evidence that the adoption of EBM is an excellent way of keeping up to date and that practitioners perform better than colleagues who rely on traditional CPD for their updates (Sackett *et al.* 2000). The practice of EBVM is a process of lifelong, self-directed problem-based learning in which caring for patients defines the need for clinically important information about patient care.

Clearly books, reviews, conferences, and meetings have their place. Indeed they provide sources of evidence in themselves and will always play a role in meeting our CPD needs, especially for our background knowledge and understanding.

### 1.5.5   *Increasing the speed of adopting the results of science*

The number of veterinary papers in the literature is expanding inexorably. Even the specialists find it hard to keep up to date and hold this knowledge in the foreground. Why wait for a second-hand version of the information to be described in a book chapter several years after the publication of the results of a clinical trial? The abstract of a trial will be available on the Internet within days of publication. The paper itself will be available online, or via the RCVS library. It is exciting and rewarding to apply our intellects and skills in delivering innovation to patients and their owners. The expression 'Science into practice' has become a dictum in human medicine.

### 1.5.6  *To better direct clinical research*

General practitioners are ultimately the consumers of clinical research. In the course of normal veterinary practice an EBVM practitioner will generate a large number of information needs, and unlike medical colleagues, will find many of them unanswered in the primary scientific literature. For some this might be a reason to dismiss the use of EBVM. However, through the use of EBVM we would soon identify the major areas of deficiency and be able to provide evidence that clinical research is needed in these areas. Those of us who perform clinical research and those who fund or direct research would benefit enormously from the input of EBVM practitioners telling us what was needed in 'the real world'.

### 1.5.7  *Ethical aspects of proof* (based upon Ramey and Rollin 2001)

Our profession has a contract with society. We are permitted to operate a 'closed shop' in providing veterinary treatment, and in return we promise to ensure certain levels of competence and adhere to certain ethical standards. We are awarded powers that are not given to the wider public, and with those powers come responsibilities. A veterinary surgeon has a moral and ethical obligation to provide treatment for which there is good evidence of its efficacy. Society expects that safe and effective treatments are provided. Therefore a salient question is 'How do we know that a treatment is safe and effective?' Within our profession, are we prepared to accept some responsibility as individuals? We can rely entirely on expert opinion or analysis, or we can be prepared to look at the primary evidence ourselves. We should attempt to ensure that an animal's condition has been accurately and objectively diagnosed, that the treatment being provided is specific for the animal condition, and that the effects of the treatment are better than merely allowing the disease to follow its natural course. The veterinary profession gains respect and trust from clients through its dedication to objective diagnosis and validation of treatments.

Society expects medical professions to be science-based, and the drug licensing regulations reflect this. Societal expectations also imply that the public expects that veterinary surgeons will use science-based canons of proof and evidence in evaluating diagnostic and treatment modalities. Even though not all standard veterinary medical treatments have been directly validated by science they are generally based upon well-established biomedical principles. We can infer or extrapolate to form an opinion (a hypothesis) based on the scientific evidence while remaining aware that this opinion does not constitute primary evidence in its own right.

### 1.5.8　*Ethical conduct in the absence of scientific evidence*
(based upon Ramey and Rollin 2001)

In our opinion, knowingly prescribing unproven treatments (i.e. those not determined to be effective by standard scientific procedures) goes against the very nature of the profession. A substantial body of scientifically sound evidence supporting conventional veterinary treatments does exist, and in cases where proof is lacking such treatments are usually based upon sound biomedical principles. It is not sufficient for a veterinary surgeon to declare that they know an unproven treatment works on the basis of his or her own personal experience. Many students are surprised to hear from an experienced practitioner that many of our patients get better in spite of our treatments rather than because of them. We should share in this humility and not believe that we have a unique instinctive insight that *guides* us to a 'new' treatment. Practitioners of EBVM are not cynical about unproven treatments but they remain sceptical about all treatments. Of course we should be ready to consider new effective treatments.

As a profession we should cast our net for effective treatments as widely as possible. However, scientific validation is the gold standard by which we can make sound judgements. The fact is that scientifically validated treatments and procedures are more likely to be safe and effective than non-validated ones and their risks are better understood than non-validated ones. Accordingly they should be the preferred option when available.

The philosophy of evidence-based medicine or practice emphasises the rigorous scientific approach to treatment decisions. In this scheme the quality of information is graded, based on the probability that the study will generate reliable conclusions and recommendations:

- Class A: evidence is best and is derived from randomised, double-blinded, placebo-controlled clinical trials
- Class B: evidence is derived from high quality clinical trials using historical controls
- Class C: evidence is from uncontrolled case series
- Class D: evidence is derived from anecdotal clinical reports, or expert opinion, or extrapolated from benchtop experiments.

It is our obligation to use the best evidence available to support a decision. It is important to keep an open mind and to consider all therapeutic possibilities (traditional and alternative) even if we cannot currently understand or explain the physiological basis for their effect. However, the science-based approach to determine the benefits and adverse effects should be maintained (Shaw 2001).

### 1.5.9   *A return to science*

We live in an age when the spectacular benefits of science are offset against a poor public perception of the scientific process. Indeed, it could be said that the public has lost faith in science. Even though we are scientifically trained, we ourselves suffer from the same problem. Many of us find it hard to comprehend the science underlying the spread of prion diseases such as BSE, and we are poorly equipped to contribute to arguments about the appropriate use of vaccination in the face of foot and mouth disease. Society generally holds us in a high regard, and yet it could be argued that our performance, as a profession, in the face of public health issues has been lacklustre. When we abandon our scientific roots, we lose our ability to evaluate evidence objectively. EBVM is a gentle reminder that our profession is still based on well-established scientific method, which should not be abandoned without good cause. One skill that appears to be in poor supply these days is the ability to understand and manage risk. The decision-making in EBVM is designed to make risk management an integral part of the process. When we are confident in this process, and communicate effectively to non-veterinary surgeons, we will be able to contribute more powerfully to discussions of public concern, both as individuals and as a profession.

### 1.5.10   *Are we ready to ask questions about our own performance?*

To end this section on a more controversial note, how many of us would like to know how good we are at what we do? We expect the competence of airline pilots to be regularly assessed, but we would probably be less happy if someone suggested it for our profession. Of course it is extremely difficult to assess veterinary performance objectively, and so the situation is unlikely to arise. On the other hand, if you were asked if you would like to be a better veterinary surgeon most of us would probably answer 'yes'. If we want to improve our performance we really need to have some measure of that performance. When we adhere to the philosophy of EBVM, we follow an explicit decision-making process, which we can subsequently review. As students of EBVM we learn about different types of decision-making process and can analyse our own decisions. Ultimately we place ourselves in a position where we can begin to ask questions about the sensitivity and specificity of our own ability to diagnose disease.

## 1.6   A more detailed description of EBVM

### 1.6.1   *The process*

'Evidence-based veterinary medicine is the use of current best evidence in making clinical decisions'.

In EBVM reduced reliance is placed upon intuition, unsystematic clinical experience, and pathophysiological assumptions as a basis for clinical decision-making, and puts the emphasis on evidence from randomised controlled trials or accurate recording of information. Meta-analyses, which statistically summarise the results from a number of randomised trials, are increasingly being used as evidence.

Evidence-based medicine is the enhancement of a clinician's traditional skills in diagnosis, treatment, prevention and related areas through the systematic framing of relevant and answerable questions and the use of mathematical estimates of probability and risk. Surveys in human medicine indicate that clinical decisions are only rarely based upon best evidence. Decision-making is often heavily influenced by anecdote (personal clinical experiences), and distortion of prevalence or outcomes. Decision-making by referring to expert opinion (eminence-based medicine) assumes evidence-based decisions, which may not always be true.

The best evidence is derived from clinically relevant research, especially from patient-centred clinical research into the accuracy and precision of diagnostic tests (including clinical examination), the power of prognostic markers, and the efficiency and safety of therapeutic and preventative regimes. New evidence from clinical research may invalidate previously accepted tests and treatments and may replace them with more powerful, more accurate, more efficacious, and safer procedures.

However, EBVM requires additional skills and an understanding of technical terms, and comes with a time cost. Skills include the ability to translate practical information needs into questions that can be answered, the skills to devise and implement an efficient strategy to obtain available scientific evidence to answer the question, the knowledge and skills required to determine which available evidence sources are the most valid and appropriate.

Veterinary clinicians are constantly faced with a range of clinical tasks associated with disease in a particular animal such as:

- interpreting diagnostic tests
- judging the efficacy of preventative or therapeutic interventions
- trying to predict the harm associated with specific therapies
- predicting the course and prognosis of the disease
- estimating the costs of the intervention.

Clinicians need to know whether their procedures and judgements are valid. The practice of EBVM identifies the clinically important information required. The process is as follows:

- information needs are transformed into a series of questions
- a search is performed for the best available evidence with which to answer the question with maximum efficiency

- the evidence obtained is critically appraised for its validity (closeness to the truth) and usefulness (clinical applicability)
- the results of this appraisal are used in clinical judgements and actions
- the outcome of the resulting decisions and actions are evaluated.

In other words EBVM leads us to restructure the problem into a series of questions that define the information needs. Sources of information are then identified. The information is then evaluated with regard to the strength of evidence it provides to support a decision. The value of the current information is then appraised for your current clinical setting.

## 1.6.2  The need for evidence

Sullivan and MacNaughton (1996) produced a subjective assessment of the sources of 'evidence' used during the consultation process performed by medical doctors. The contributions from four sources of evidence identified were estimated for each part of the consultation process. This is shown in table 1.2.

**Table 1.2**  Sources of evidence used during consultation.

|  | Undergraduate studies | Experience | Scientific evidence | Wider literature |
|---|---|---|---|---|
| Taking a history | ++ | +++ | + | ++ |
| Clinical examination and diagnosis | ++ | +++ | +++ | + |
| Treatment/prognosis/control | ++ | +++ | +++ | ++ |
| Explaining the diagnosis to the owner | + | +++ | + | +++ |
| Make effective use of consultation | + | +++ | +++ | +++ |

Within each component of the consultation process a number of sources of evidence were used with some sources used more frequently than others. It is clear that scientific evidence had an important contribution to make as a source of evidence.

However, it must also be accepted that whatever source of evidence is used it must be valid. This has been stated more forcefully by Bonnett (1998). 'An understanding of basic pathophysiological mechanisms of disease is necessary but is not sufficient grounds for decision making in clinical medicine. As important as clinical acumen, experience and judgement are, we must move beyond dependence on anecdote, personal experience, and expert opinion towards validated evidence-based medicine'.

### 1.6.3   *Other sources of information and evidence*

If scientific evidence is unavailable, clinical experience may provide the only evidence. However, memory is selective and not unbiased. Therefore systematic, reliable, and reproducible recording of observations provides better information than unquantified experience and intuition. Systematic, accurate, data recording and appraisal of this information is part of EBVM. Good examples include dairy farm recording of lameness, fertility and mastitis.

## 1.7   EBM in human medicine

In human medicine there is now an established methodology called evidence-based medicine (EBM). There are six journals publishing articles related to this topic, countless textbooks in every discipline of medicine, numerous training courses at post-graduate level, and an ever increasing number of medical schools with EBM as part of curricula.

The growth of interest and development of the principles of EBM in human medicine have been fuelled by:

- the daily need for valid information about diagnosis, prognosis, therapy and prevention
- the inadequacy of traditional sources because they are out of date, frequently wrong, ineffective or too overwhelming in their volume and too variable in their validity for practical clinical use
- the disparity between our diagnostic skills and clinical judgement which increase with experience and our up-to-date knowledge and overall clinical performance which declines
- the recognition that allocation of time working on a patient's problems may be better served by spending less time on clinical procedures and more time in finding and appraising evidence to support clinical judgements.

Developments that have allowed this situation to change are:

- the development of search strategies for efficiently tracking down and appraising evidence (for its validity and relevance)
- the creation of systematic reviews and concise summaries
- the creation of evidence-based journals of secondary publication
- the creation of information systems to allow fast access
- the identification and application of effective strategies for lifelong learning and for improving clinical performance.

## 1.8   EBM in veterinary medicine

EBVM and EBM are very closely related and differ mainly in the availability of evidence. In veterinary science the literature base is much smaller; restricting sources of information from systematic research may omit other useful sources of information which may be difficult to validate but on which a weighting can be subjectively applied so that due emphasis can be given to it. The human interpretation of EBM provides an ideal goal to aim at but is too narrow in its definition for veterinary science. As EBM developed much earlier than EBVM an understanding of EBM is instructive in looking forward in the development of EBVM.

The main differences between the practice of EBM in veterinary medicine and human medicine lie in the emphasis we necessarily place in evaluating poorer sources of evidence. The medical practitioner may dismiss a report of a single case as mere anecdote, whereas the veterinary practitioner may be grateful to have found a single published reference. In EBVM, because our decision-making process will be complicated by a variety of evidence, we place emphasis on understanding how we make decisions to accommodate greater levels of uncertainty. As veterinary surgeons we are placed in situations in which we handle more risk. The better management of this risk is a skill that we, our patients, and our clients can benefit from.

There is an increasing body of opinion that EBVM is vital to the future development of the profession, and recent textbooks are now describing the concept (Bonnett 1998, Polzin *et al.* 2000, Radostits *et al.* 2000). The lack of methodically performed, rigorous, large-scale clinical studies in veterinary medicine has been recognized by the Comparative Clinical Science Panel of the Medical Research Council. This organisation aims to provide a strategic focus for veterinary research, especially clinical research, to expand the evidence base for the practice of veterinary medicine.

A serious movement towards EBVM will require that a large body of high quality patient-centred research be available to veterinary surgeons willing, and able, to access and critically appraise the quality and applicability of clinical trials. The relatively small size of the database in veterinary medicine may impede the application of EBVM but there is now a new emphasis on the importance of randomised controlled trials.

One database search for evidence regarding the treatment of lymphoma in dogs in 2000 found 60 publications but few were designed to address important therapeutic issues. A search of the human literature, using the same key words produced 5400 studies many with results from randomized placebo-controlled trials.

EBVM has been slow to develop as an independent discipline. A literature database search in 2001 found 5822 references to EBM but only 17 references to EBVM (Roper 2001). There are no post-graduate training courses, no specific journals and, at the time of writing, no dedicated textbooks. Cambridge Veterinary School has a short undergraduate course on the subject but this topic has yet to be established in undergraduate veterinary curricula in the UK. Although clinical students are encouraged to identify the best current sources of information, the practice of EBM, the skill levels and the access to resources are largely unmeasured.

## 1.9   Are we already practising EBVM?

A simple way of assessing your own performance as an EBVM practitioner would be to answer the following questions:

- Do I identify and prioritize the problems to be solved (information needs)?
- Do I perform a competent and complete examination to establish the likelihood of alternative diagnoses?
- Do I have an accurate knowledge of disease manifestations, the sign sensitivities and specificities, and the frequency of occurrence of different combinations of clinical signs within a disease(s)?
- Do I search for the missing information?
- Do I appraise the information in terms of scientific validity?
- Do I understand the scientific terms such as specificity and sensitivity, which will enable me to interpret the information provided?
- Do I have the resources to access the Internet?
- Am I aware of the veterinary information databases?
- Am I aware of the veterinary decision support systems that are available?
- Is the application of new information scientifically justified, and intuitively sensible for this situation?
- Do I explain the pros and cons of the different opinions taking into account the different utilities to the owner?

Even avid EBVM practitioners will answer 'not always' to some of these questions but an awareness of our deficiencies is the first step to remedying them.

## 1.10   EBVM case studies

The purpose of these case studies is to highlight how evidence-based approaches can contribute towards decision-making in clinical practice. They also illustrate that there is a need to critically appraise the evidence being presented. Are the conclusions valid based upon the experimental design and the statistical analysis used?

### 1.10.1   *Small animals: megavoltage radiotherapy of nasal tumours in dogs*

A dog is presented with chronic sneezing, occasional unilateral epistaxis and nasal discharge. Histopathology indicates that this is a nasal squamous cell carcinoma. At a recent CPD event megavoltage radiotherapy was proposed as the best current primary therapy. The owner wishes to know if the animal will be cured following treatment, if there will be any side effects, if the clinical signs are likely to resolve, and what the survival time is likely to be.

You perform a Medline search online (using Pubmed) and find a retrospective study undertaken on 56 dogs treated for nasal tumours by megavoltage radiotherapy by Mellanby *et al.* (2002) published in the *Veterinary Record*. In your flat upstairs you find the issue and read the paper. You are able to address the client's concerns from the information contained in the paper.

The paper reports that a median survival time after the last dose was 212 days. The 1-year and 2-year survival rates were 45% and 15%, respectively. Fifty dogs were euthanased because of the recurrence of the initial clinical signs. At the end of the 4 weeks of treatment: of the 45 dogs presenting with sneezing 40% (18) no longer sneezed and a further 26 (58%) had improved; of the 37 dogs presenting with epistaxis 27 (73%) no longer had epistaxis and 10 (27%) had improved; of the 33 dogs presenting with nasal discharge 21% no longer had a discharge and nine (36%) had a reduced discharge. Mild acute radiation side effects (erythema, mucositis and regional alopecia) were observed in the majority of dogs but long-term radiation side effects were rare (one dog).

No veterinary surgeon will provide categoric promises on the basis of this information. However, an educated, or well-informed client might be interested in the basis upon which their questions were answered. Some clients will be entirely focused on the outcome for their animal and place their trust (and the consequential responsibility) in your hands. In this case, while the client may not wish to be aware of this evidence, it increases your confidence in accepting this trust and shouldering the responsibility.

### 1.10.2 *Farm animals: restocking after foot and mouth disease*

A farmer is restocking after compulsory slaughter as a contiguous property in the UK foot and mouth 2001 outbreak. After reading advice leaflets on biosecurity and restocking, the farmer is interested in testing his new dairy herd of 200 dairy cattle at the farm of origin for tuberculosis and Johne's disease. He asks you how good the tests are.

The test for TB is the single intra-dermal comparative test using *Mycobacterium bovis* purified protein derivative (PPD) and *M. avium* PPD.

The test for Johne's could be the agar-gel immunodiffusion test (AGID), the complement fixation test (CFT), bacteriological culture of faeces, and the enzyme-linked immunoabsorbent assay (ELISA) all offered by the Veterinary Laboratories Agency (VLA) in the UK.

You do a Medline search and you identify papers which seem to be of interest. One is a paper entitled 'Pathogenesis and diagnosis of infections with *Myco-*

*bacterium bovis* in cattle' by Morrison *et al.* (2000) published in the *Veterinary Record*.

This review described a large study in a comparable population reporting a sensitivity of about 90%. The sensitivity is the percentage of the truly infected animals correctly identified by the test. Studies on the specificity of the test indicate a value in excess of 99%. The specificity is the percentage of the truly uninfected animals that are correctly identified by the test.

The high specificity indicates that false positives are unlikely. However, the failure to detect 10% of infected animals with a single test is some cause for concern. The farmer will be looking for a test where a negative test is likely to produce a TB free herd. You are able to indicate how confident the farmer can be in the results.

You do a Medline search and find a paper (Smith and Slenning 2000) which provides you with the sensitivity and specificity of the four tests of interest designed to detect Johne's disease in the subclinical stages of the disease. On credit card payment of $30 you obtain the full text paper via the Internet.

|  | Sensitivity | Specificity | Cost (VLA 2002/2003) |
|---|---|---|---|
| AGID | 0.35 | 1.00 | £5.95 |
| CFT | 0.25 | 0.95 | £13.20 |
| Bacteriological culture | 0.45 | 1.00 | £25.95 |
| ELISA | 0.45 | 0.99 | £5.95 |

From this information the ELISA test would be the most useful screening test. But the farmer must be aware that only 45% of subclinical animals that are truly infected will be detected by the test and that 55% will go undetected.

### 1.10.3   *Horses: efficiency of prednisolone for the treatment of heaves (COPD)*

You are presented with a stabled horse with acute heaves (COPD). You decide that a short course of corticosteroid is the most appropriate treatment in the short term. You are aware that oral prednisolone has been recommended by several recently published textbooks and that the tablets would be easier for the owner to administer. Prednisolone is also thought to present less risk of inducing laminitis. The owner asks you if it is as effective as 'the injection' (i.e. dexamethasone).

You have never questioned this and decide to check the literature. Following a Medline search on Pubmed you identify a recent study entitled 'Efficiency of three corticosteroids for the treatment of heaves' by Robinson *et al.* (2002) . This study used a cross-over design with nine horses with heaves. There was a negative control (no treatment), and a positive control (dexamethasone i.v.). Dexamethasone rapidly relieved airway obstruction in the heaves-affected horses. Oral prednisolone had no immediate effect and even after 10 days treatment the improvement was not statistically significantly different from the negative control. The authors conclude that these results call into question the efficacy of oral prednisolone in the treatment of heaves.

## 1.11 How this book is organised

### 1.11.1 The aims and objectives of this book

This book aims to explain what EBVM is, and how it can be applied to veterinary practice.

By reading this book you should achieve the following objectives:

- understand the process of diagnosis and the output of clinical diagnostic decision support systems
- know how to transform information needs into a series of clinical questions that can be answered from the literature and other information sources
- know how to search for best available external evidence
- know how to critically appraise the evidence for its validity and importance
- know how to apply it in clinical practice.

This will optimise:

- achieving a diagnosis
- estimating a prognosis
- deciding on the best treatment
- patient welfare
- prevention and control of the disease.

The primary concerns of this book are the quality of clinical information and its correct interpretation. We have not written this book for those who do clinical research but for those who depend upon it. The structure reflects this. The book is organised primarily according to the clinical questions encountered when veterinary surgeons are presented with a disease problem.

### 1.11.2 Outline of the structure of this book

The book is organised into the following chapters.

- Chapter 2: Turning information needs into questions. Identifying information needs and converting these needs into scientific questions that may be answered from the literature.

- Chapter 3: Sources of information. This chapter describes the different sources of information that are available to the veterinary surgeon.
- Chapter 4: Searching for evidence. This chapter focuses upon searching the Internet and in particular using the Pubmed website to search the Medline database of abstracts, and explains the use of search strategies to find papers on diagnosis, therapy, prognosis, and aetiology.
- Chapter 5: Research studies. The aim of this chapter is to enable the reader to understand the strengths and weaknesses of the different types of studies and thereby learn to identify the studies of greatest relevance to their own questions.
- Chapter 6: Appraising the evidence. The aim of this chapter is to provide basic guidelines for determining the validity and relevance of clinical studies. This evaluation is obtained by answering the questions 'Is it true?' and 'Is it relevant to my question/patient?'.
- Chapter 7: Diagnosis. The aim of this chapter is to present the methods of data collection and clinical reasoning used in the diagnostic process so that the process can be made explicit.
- Chapter 8: Clinical diagnostic decision support systems. In this chapter the different methods used in clinical diagnostic decision support systems and how these systems can be evaluated in terms of their diagnostic ability are described.
- Chapter 9: Decision analysis, models and economics as evidence. This chapter explains how decision analysis can be used to make decisions under conditions of uncertainty. It also explains how models can be used in the decision-making process and how economics can be used as a decision tool.
- Chapter 10: EBVM: Education and future needs. This final chapter examines the current and future needs to support EBVM and explains how clinical audits may become an EBM tool in veterinary science.

## References and further reading

Badenoch, D. and Heneghan, C. (2002) *Evidence-based Medicine Toolkit.* BMJ Books, London.

Bonnett, B. (1998) *Evidence-based Medicine: critical evaluation of new and existing therapies in complementary and alternative veterinary medicine principles and practice.* Mosby, London, chapter 2.

Gross, R. (2001) Decisions and evidence in medical practice. In *Veterinary Clinical Examination and Diagnosis* (eds Radostits, O.M., Mayhew, I.G.J. and Houston, D.M.). W.B. Saunders, London.

Keene, W.B. (2000) Editorial: towards evidence-based veterinary medicine. *Journal of Veterinary Internal Medicine* **14**, 118–19.

Macon, A., Smith, H., White, P. and Field, J. (1998) General practitioners' perceptions of the route to evidence based medicine: a questionnaire survey. *British Medical Journal* **316**, 361–5.

Mellanby, R.J., Stevenson, R.K., Herrtage, M.E., White, R.A.S. and Dobson, J.M. (2002)

Long-term outcome of 56 dogs with nasal tumours treated with four doses of radiation at intervals of 7 days. *Veterinary Record* **151**, 253–7.

Morrison, W.I., Bourne, F.J., Cox, D.R., Donnelly, C.A., Gettinby, G., McInerney, J.P. and Woodroffe, R. (2000) Pathogenesis and diagnosis of infections with *Mycobacterium bovis* in cattle. *Veterinary Record* **146**, 236–42.

Polzin, D.J., Land, E., Walter, P. and Klausner, J. (2000) From journal to patient: evidence-based medicine. In *Kirk's Current Veterinary Therapy XIII Small Animal Practice* (ed. Bonagura, J.D.). W.B. Saunders Company, London.

Radostits, O.M., Tyler, J.W. and Mayhew, I.G.J. (2000) Making a diagnosis. In *Veterinary Clinical Examination and Diagnosis* (eds Radostits, O.M., Mayhew, I.G.J. and Houston, D.M.). W.B. Saunders, London, chapter 2.

Ramey D.W. and Rollin, B.E. (2001) Ethical aspects of proof and 'alternative' therapies. *JAVMA* **218** (3), 343–6.

Robinson, N.E., Jackson, C., Jefcoat, A., Berney, C., Peroni, D. and Derksen, F.J. (2002) Efficiency of three corticosteroids for the treatment of heaves. *Equine Veterinary Journal* **34** (1), 17–22.

Roper, T. (2001) EAHIL Workshop, Alghero, 7–9 June, www.rcvs.org.uk

Sackett, D.L., Straus, S.E., Richardson, S.W. and Rosenberg, W. (2000) *Evidence-based Medicine: How to Practice and Teach EBM*. Churchill Livingstone, Edinburgh.

Shaughnessy, A.F., Slawson, D.C. and Bennett J.H. (1994) Becoming an information master: a guide book to the medical information jungle. *Journal of Family Practice* **39**, 489–99.

Shaw, D. (2001) Veterinary medicine is science-based: an absolute or an option? *Canadian Veterinary Journal* **42**, 333–4.

Smith, R. (1996) Information in practice: What clinical information do doctors need? *British Medical Journal* **313**, 1062–8.

Smith, R.D. and Slenning, B.D. (2000) Decision analysis: dealing with uncertainty in diagnostic testing. *Preventive Veterinary Medicine* **45** (1–2), 139–62.

Sullivan, F.M. and MacNaughton, R.J. (1996) Evidence in consultations: interpreted and individualised. *Lancet* **348**, 941–3.

Veterinary Marketing Association (2001) Vetstream Ltd UK Online Publication. Issue **8**, 1.

## Review questions

Choose the best single answer for the following questions. Answers on page 204

**1  Which of the following is the best definition of EBVM?**

 (a) Evidence-based veterinary medicine is the conscientious, explicit and judicious use of current best evidence in making clinical decisions
 (b) Evidence-based medicine is a method used by experts in referral centre
 (c) Evidence-based veterinary medicine is a literature search to find papers on a topic of interest.

**2  Usefulness of medical information can be defined as**

 (a) How often you use it
 (b) Outcome – Time cost
 (c) Usefulness of medical information $= \dfrac{\text{relevance} \times \text{validity}}{\text{work to access}}$

**3  Evidence-based veterinary medicine is now more possible than ever before because:**

 (a) Textbooks are more rapidly updated
 (b) Information technology enables rapid searching for information
 (c) There is now an abundance of published literature
 (d) Clients are willing to pay for it.

**4  Evidence-based veterinary medicine is based upon:**

 (a) Information published in a veterinary journal
 (b) Information that has been scientifically validated
 (c) Any source of information
 (d) Personal experience.

**5  To practise evidence-based veterinary medicine requires:**

 (a) A new set of skills which includes computer searching and scientific paper evaluation
 (b) Time but no new skills
 (c) More traditional CPD.

# 2

# TURNING
# INFORMATION
# NEEDS INTO
# QUESTIONS

The aim of this chapter is to explain how clinical problems can be translated into questions which may be answered using sources of information that are available to practitioners.

At the end of this chapter the reader should be able to address the following three questions:

- Have I established that I have all the information required to optimise the patient care?
- If I need further information have I formulated the problem into a question that can be answered?
- Do I understand the formal scientific terminology that I will need to answer the question?

23

## 2.1   Introduction

One of the hardest steps in practising EBVM may be the translation of a clinical problem (as presented in the consulting room) into an answerable clinical question. These answers must be achieved in a sensible timeframe, and at a reasonable cost, in terms of the time and effort involved.

The first important concept is 'Knowing what you don't know'. It may not be obvious to a busy clinician that in order to provide the best patient care there is a need for additional information and an assessment of how good the evidence to support the information is. Once the clinical problem has been identified one of the hardest steps in practising EBVM is the translation of clinical problems into an answerable clinical question for which a search for evidence can be made. The question may be about the optimal diagnostic approach, therapeutic strategy or prognosis. The definition and structure of an appropriate question is crucial if the search for appropriate evidence is to be successful. The question should define the clinical problem using scientific terminology that will identify the evidence required, and lead us to the most efficient search strategy to locate that evidence.

## 2.2   Refining clinical questions so that evidence can be found

A clinical question may have many forms as follows.

### 2.2.1   *Is this a good treatment for a disease?*

An answerable question would be:

- What is the probability of a cure with the treatment compared with an alternative standard therapy in a patient that has the disease in a population like mine?

### 2.2.2   *How good is a test?*

What will a result positive or negative test really mean? In other words, how confidently can I rely on the results?

The ways we can evaluate or appraise a paper describing a diagnostic test are described in Chapter 4. Firstly we need to know two measures of the test's performance:

- How frequently is the test positive in animals with the disease? (the sensitivity of the test)

- How frequently is the test negative in animals without the disease? (the specificity of the test)

From these and the pre-test probability of disease (the prevalence) we can derive the post-test probability of disease (the chance of my patient having the disease if testing positive, and the chance of my patient having the disease if testing negative).

## 2.3   Four main elements of a well-formed clinical question (PICO)

The four main elements of a good clinical question can be remembered from the mnemonic **PICO**, **P**atient, **I**ntervention, **C**omparison, and **O**utcome.

### 2.3.1   *Patient or problem*

How would I categorise the patient and/or the problem. This may include signalment such as age or breed, the primary problem, and the population to which the affected animals belong.

This will help identify studies or evidence for similar populations of patient, e.g. chronic weight loss in an middle-aged cross-bred dog.

### 2.3.2   *The diagnostic or therapeutic intervention, prognostic factor or exposure*

Which main intervention, prognostic factor or exposure are you considering? What do you want to do for the patient, e.g. prescribe a drug, order a test, or perform surgery? What factor may influence the prognosis of the patient, e.g. age or co-existing problems? What kind of environment is the animal exposed to, e.g. will zinc sulphate foot baths reduce the prevalence/incidence of digital dermatitis in cattle?

### 2.3.3   *Comparison of interventions (if appropriate or required)*

What is the main alternative to compare to the intervention? Are you trying to decide between two drugs, or between a drug and no medication, or between two diagnostic tests? In order to identify the comparison, a useful approach is to consider what you would do if the intervention was not performed. This may be nothing or a standard care protocol.

For example, how would zinc sulphate foot baths compare to oxytetracycline foot baths in the treatment of digital dermatitis in cattle?

### 2.3.4   The outcome

What outcome is important, to the patient, and the owner? What is an appropriate time frame for the response? This may require a cost–benefit analysis based upon economics or welfare. What can you hope to accomplish, measure, improve or affect? What are you trying to do for the patient, obtain a cure, prevent deterioration, reduce chronic pain, or increase function?

For example, is there a reduction in the annual incidence of digital dermatitis in the herd with the monthly use of zinc sulphate (as opposed to oxytetracycline treatment)?

## 2.4   Categorising the type of question being asked

It is useful to categorise the type of question you are asking:

- epidemiological risk factors
- diagnostic process
- clinical examination
- differential diagnosis
- diagnostic tests/further investigations
- treatment
- harm
- prognosis
- control and prevention.

## 2.5   Prioritising the questions

When you have more questions than time consider:

- Which question is the most important to the animal's welfare?
- Which question is the most feasible to answer in the time available?
- Which question is most interesting to you?
- Which question are you most likely to encounter repeatedly during the course of your work?
- Which question has the lowest time cost but the greatest cost/clinical benefit?

## 2.6   Checklist of information needs

Some of the terminology used in these checklists is described in other chapters (mainly in Chapter 6).

## 2.6.1   *Epidemiological risk factors*

These are risk factors that determine the occurrence and distribution of disease in a population.

- What is the incubation period?
- How long can the organism survive outside the host?
- What factors influence this survival?
- What is the method of spread?
- How contagious is the organism?
- Is there a carrier state?
- Are all carriers excreting the organism?
- Is the carrier state lifelong?
- Are all infected animals clinically affected?
- Is there a screening test?
- What is the sensitivity and specificity of the test?
- How many animals do I need to test to confirm the aetiology at a given prevalence level?
- How long does it take for the serological antibodies to rise following infection?
- How long do the antibodies persist for following infection?
- Is there a licensed vaccine?
- Are serological antibodies an indication of protection?
- How good is the protection afforded by the vaccine?
- How often does the vaccine have to be given?
- Can the vaccine be given at any age and stage of pregnancy?
- Does the vaccine affect fertility/function?
- Can the vaccine be used in the face of an outbreak?
- How quickly and what level of protection is provided?
- Can vaccinated animals be detected?
- Can vaccinated animals be distinguished from naturally infected animals?

## 2.6.2   **Diagnostic process**

- What is the sensitivity and specificity of the clinical signs for each disease?
- What is the prevalence of potential diseases in your area?
- What is the probability of a disease given the presence of a clinical sign?
- What is the probability of disease given the absence of a sign?
- What is known about the pathophysiology of the disease?
- What are the risk factors for these potential diseases and are they operating in the local environment so that the prevalences locally may need to be revised?

*Decision support systems*

- Did it contain all the potential diseases?
- Is the information about the diseases accurate?
- Do you understand the methodology being used?
- Is the methodology flawed?
- Has the system been validated using real cases from comparable populations?
- Have specificity and sensitivity been defined?
- Were the differential diagnosis ranked?
- If so, how would the ranking change if you considered rank by:
  seriousness
  probability
  treatability?

*Diagnostic tests/further investigations*

- Was the population used the same as mine?
- Do you know the accuracy of the test?
- Do you know the specificity of the test?
- Do you know the sensitivity of the test?
- Do you know the pre-test odds before the test?
- Do you know the likelihood ratio of a positive result?
- Do you know the likelihood ratio of a negative test?
- Are the tests being performed by a laboratory with strict quality control?
- Are the normal ranges used for interpretation meaningful?
- Are the tests confirming or trying to rule out differential diagnoses?
- Will the test, irrespective of the result, provide discriminatory information?

*Methodology when considering the use of a test*

- Find the positive likelihood ratio and negative likelihood ratio for the test.
- Estimate the pre-test probability of the disease in the patient.
- Apply the likelihood ratio to the pre-test probabilities.
- Consider the additional discriminatory information that is being provided and how invasive/expensive the test is.
- Make a decision to perform the test, or not, in consultation with the owner.

### 2.6.3   Treatment

What measures are useful to provide evidence about treatments? Evidence may be required to validate:

- efficacy
- dose

- frequency
- length of treatment
- combinations of drugs
- licensed (cascade considerations)
- costs
- harm caused by treatment versus harm caused by disease
- residues/withdrawal times.

It would be useful to be able to provide the patient with a probability that the treatment will be successful.

Effective treatments operate by improving outcomes of a disease. Such an improvement should be considered in two ways:

- Increasing the likelihood of a good outcome (e.g. increased survival)
- Decreasing the likelihood of a bad outcome (e.g. reduced mortality).

Terms to consider when asking questions about treatment or harm caused by treatments are (see Chapter 6, Section 2):

- Absolute risk reduction
- Relative risk reduction
- Number needed to treat
- Number needed to harm
- What will the impact, harm, or improvement be for my patient?

### 2.6.4   Harm/aetiology

What do I know about the risk factors (see Chapter 6, Section 4)? Useful parameters to characterise harm are:

- relative risk, and odds ratios
- number needed to harm (NNH).

Does the reduction in consequences of the additional risk warrant the cost of reducing or removing exposure?

### 2.6.5   Prognosis

With any clinical problem always ask the question 'does the awareness of the likelihoods of the various outcomes over time help the owner/veterinary surgeon make important decisions about the future of the animal?'. Outlined below are some of the factors and information needs that you may wish to consider when providing a prognosis.

*Impact on the patient and the owner*

Successful operation may leave the animal disfigured or dysfunctional, even though the problem was cured, e.g. bone tumour of the jaw, lameness in a horse.

*Prognostic indicators*

> Likelihood ratios can be determined for particular features of a disease, which have a prognostic value. They can therefore be considered in the same way as a diagnostic test (see Chapter 6, Section 5).

*Outcomes*

> The outcomes and the likelihood of these outcomes will be dependent on which treatment strategy is used.

*Timing*

> The timeframes of the important outcomes including when they occur and how long they last are desirable components of a prognosis. Owners benefit from knowing when an outcome can be expected, particularly if the condition is progressive, debilitating, and invariably fatal. The pattern of survival over time, and the quality of life over time, are important considerations in a fatal disease.
>
> The risk of the outcome over time can be expressed:
>
> - as a percentage of survival at a particular point in time?
> - as a median survival time (the length of time by which 50% of study patients have had the outcome)?
> - as a survival curve that depicts at each point in time the proportion (expressed as a percentage) of the original study sample who have not yet had a specified outcome?

### 2.6.6   *Control (risk reduction) and prevention (risk avoidance)*

> - Have I identified all the important risk factors associated with the epidemiology of the disease?
> - Do the animals exposed to the risk have a higher incidence of outcome compared with animals that are not exposed?
> - Is there an increase in the outcome by exposure to the risk? Does the reduction in risk justify the cost/effort of removing or reducing the exposure by vaccination and/or vaccination?

## 2.7   Potential pitfalls in constructing questions

> There are a number of potential pitfalls that need to be considered when translating clinical problems into well-constructed clinical questions.

### 2.7.1   Complexity of the questions

There may be just too many questions generated from a single clinical case, or the case itself may be too complicated. We have to learn to prioritise the questions and leave some questions unanswered. We look for answers to the questions that are most relevant to this particular case and also those questions for which we are likely to obtain an answer.

### 2.7.2   The need for sufficient background knowledge

It can be difficult to decide if the breed is an important factor in a condition without first knowing about breed predispositions. Similarly, animals with concurrent disease, or already on medication, may or may not be important in framing questions. Seek the opinions of specialist or experienced colleagues in helping formulate the question, without necessarily deferring to their opinion as the only answer to the question.

### 2.7.3   More questions than time

For the average veterinary practitioner there will always be more questions than time. During a 15-minute consultation many clients will hope, if not expect, to receive a diagnosis, treatment, and prognosis for their animal. Within the medical world common clinical questions are addressed as CATs (critically appraised topics – see Chapter 3, Section 8). Within a practice the work of looking for the answers to common clinical questions could be shared among individuals, and collated for practice use. The search for recently produced evidence and the discussion of its results provides an excellent way of making CPD time both enjoyable, and productive.

## 2.8   Realistic targets for veterinary practice

Asking the right questions is the best way to start practising EBVM. It isn't possible to embark on a fully evidenced-based approach starting with your next case. A realistic first step is to look at common interventions used in the clinic (which are currently answering clinical questions), and to readdress those questions. What regimes do you use for post-operative analgesia? What are your vaccine recommendations? What are your standard dermatological work-ups? For all these common clinical situations there are questions to be asked, and evidence for providing the best answers.

## 2.9   Evidence of quality control

It is useful to question the evidence that supports the assumption that laboratory reports are correct when clinical pathology results are outsourced. Quality control and quality assessment are being recorded and analysed by organisations such as the National External Quality Assessment Scheme (NEQAS) for clinical pathology. This provides evidence to establish best practice for this area of diagnostic work. If a third party interpretation is used during diagnosis, what is the evidence to indicate the level of expertise of the person providing that interpretation? Are biopsy reports coming from qualified pathologists such as Members of the Royal College of Pathologists? When referring an animal to a specialist practice, what is the evidence to support the level of expertise being offered by the practice? Within our own practices, what is the evidence establishing the quality of our in-house laboratory results? Do we appraise our radiography standards to provide evidence that they are suitable for diagnostic use. Although the licensing process requires the submission of evidence on safety and efficacy this information is not readily available for detailed scrutiny.

Quality assurance is becoming established in agriculture, education and medicine. While we may not welcome the unthinking dogma that may accompany such schemes, there are clear benefits to be obtained in the quality of care for our patients from a measured introduction of the concept into our own practices.

## Further reading

Badenoch, D. and Heneghan, C. (2002) *Evidence-based Medicine Toolkit.* BMJ Books, London, p. 2.

McGovern, D.P.B., Valori, R.M., Summerskill, W.S.M. and Levi, M. (2001) *Key Topics in Evidence-based Medicine.* BIOS Scientific Publications Ltd, Oxford, p. 11.

## Review questions

Answers on page 204

**1**  *The most useful question regarding a test is:*

    (a)  What is the accuracy of the test?
    (b)  What is the specificity?
    (c)  What is the sensitivity?
    (d)  What are the specificity and sensitivity?

**2**  *Four main elements in devising a question are:*

    (a)  Defining: the patient or problem, the diagnostic or therapeutic intervention prognostic factor or exposure, comparison of interventions and the outcome
    (b)  Defining: the age of the animal, vaccination status, breed and time of onset
    (c)  Speed, accuracy, applicability and brevity.

**3**  *Which of the following categories are most useful to identify information needs?*

    (a)  Epidemiological risk factors
    (b)  Diagnostic process
    (c)  Treatment
    (d)  Harm
    (e)  Prognosis
    (f)  Control and prevention
    (g)  All of the above categories.

**4**  *Which of the following provides evidence of quality control?*

    (a)  The automatic biochemical analyser is serviced on time
    (b)  Radiographs are developed using an automatic developer
    (c)  The clinical pathology laboratory is part of an independent quality control audit scheme.

**5**  *Questions about prognosis should include:*

    (a)  The timeframes of the important outcomes including when they occur and how long they last
    (b)  The median survival time
    (c)  The pattern of survival over time, and the quality of life over time
    (d)  All of the above.

# 3

# SOURCES OF
# INFORMATION

The aim of this chapter is to indicate the range of different information resources that are available to veterinary clinicians from which evidence can be obtained.

On completing this chapter readers should:

- Appreciate the difference between foreground and background knowledge
- Be reminded of the traditional sources of veterinary information
- Know some of the sources of veterinary information available on the Internet.

## 3.1   Introduction

Clinicians do not need this book to advise them to consult respected colleagues or that the scientific practice of veterinary medicine is built upon a knowledge of the primary literature found in journals. No single source of evidence is ever going to be sufficient for our day-to-day needs, and new sources of information are developing rapidly. However, the aim of this chapter is to provide an overview of the potential sources of information with an emphasis on resources available via the Internet. To this end readers will need to have, or to develop, the skills necessary to use a personal computer, and to be able to browse the Internet using a web browser. Competence in the use of computers represents a useful life skill and, with time, we will take computers and the Internet for granted, as everyday tools for work in almost any area of endeavour.

## 3.2   Background and foreground knowledge

Background knowledge refers to the fundamental understanding of a topic and correlates largely with an individual's experience. A veterinary student might have a limited knowledge about the management of diabetes. He or she might need to refer to textbooks, attend lectures and observe cases before becoming competent in dealing with routine cases. If that student goes on to specialise in internal medicine or endocrinology that background knowledge may become profound. The knowledge we acquire must be based on valid evidence as much as possible but when it becomes a fundamental part of our understanding of a disease or treatment it is classified as background knowledge.

Foreground knowledge on the other hand refers to those bits of evidence that answer specific, focused questions. Such questions may arise from a single clinical case, and may be unique to a particular patient. Should questions arise over the use of newly emerging drug therapies the textbooks may well be old and out of date; they may be based on opinion rather than recently published clinical trial data. In such a case foreground knowledge is required which is most likely to come from skilled appraisal of the primary literature.

With time, foreground knowledge rapidly changes and may ultimately become background knowledge but it is required to provide the best possible care for individual patients. Both inexperienced clinicians and experts will need to acquire background knowledge when faced with new clinical situations (an unfamiliar species, an exotic disease, etc.). It would be inappropriate to be searching for research papers to meet our information needs in such a case when expert colleagues or textbooks are available.

## 3.3   Hierarchy of evidence

The hierarchy of evidence is a spectrum of potential sources with the source most likely to provide the best evidence at the top. The arrangement of the list will depend on the clinical question being asked. Randomised controlled trials are best for examining interventions; cohort and case–control studies are useful for addressing questions about causation. Evidence of a more anecdotal nature such as case reports will lie towards the base.

In our desire to be methodical and systematic it is important to realise that a study where $n = 1$ may be the most important piece of evidence when the experimental subject is the animal in front of us. However compelling the evidence in a paper may be for a new treatment, if a treatment worked in the past for our patient, this is good evidence not to change it.

The hierarchy of evidence in the human medical world would look something like figure 3.1. They are in a position to largely ignore any evidence other than that which appears in the medical literature. Veterinary surgeons on the other hand need to make many more decisions on where to place evidence in their hierarchies. The opinion of the pathologist, who is a Member of the Royal College of Pathologists, is probably of more value than a less well-qualified individual. A case report in peer-reviewed journal may be poorer evidence than the experience of a colleague in our own practice.

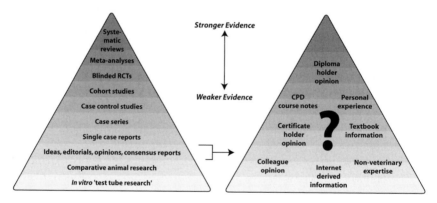

**Fig. 3.1**   An illustration of the hierarchy of evidence. The pyramid on the right indicates the difficulty in ranking much of the evidence used in clinical veterinary work

Considering the hierarchy of evidence that might apply to our case helps in the search for evidence. We want to start looking at the top, because that is where we will get the best evidence. We must try to avoid the temptation to look at sources just because they are convenient or accessible. However, much of the evidence we are forced to use as veterinary surgeons sits near the base of the pyramid. As figure 3.1 suggests, there are no generic, or absolute rules for positioning evidence in the hierarchy for all cases. We should nonetheless attempt a judgement of the relative strengths of the evidence used in each individual case.

## 3.4   Important traditional information resources

As has already been stated, there is no single source of evidence which can meet our every need, and we should be aware of the wide variety of repositories available.

### 3.4.1   *Journals*

At the heart of EBVM is the pursuit of primary evidence upon which to make health-care decisions on our patients. The single most important source of such information is from peer-reviewed papers that appear in journals. Indeed much of the rest of this book is directly or indirectly about how to use the veterinary scientific literature. The peer review process has evolved as a fundamental quality control process in the publication of scientific papers. In short, each published paper is reviewed anonymously by two or more suitably qualified scientists who work in that field. The reviewers are unpaid and impartial. Poor papers may still sometimes get published but it generally ensures that the results and conclusions of published papers can be believed. Before we can apply the information contained within such papers to our own clinical practice we do need to find the relevant papers, and be able to interpret and appraise the evidence. These tasks are covered in Chapters 4, 5 and 6.

Although scientific journals have been available throughout the history of veterinary medicine there are two recent major developments described in this chapter. The first is the availability of online indexes to enable us to search for articles of interest (introduced below), and the second, is the availability of a large number of journals also via the Internet.

At the time of writing, members of the Royal College of Veterinary Surgeons (RCVS) can access the following websites providing full text access to journals online:

- www.blackwell-synergy.com
     *Anatomia, Histologia, Embryologia:*
     *Journal of Veterinary Medicine Series C*
     *Ethology*
     *Journal of Animal Breeding and Genetics*
     *Journal of Animal Physiology and Animal Nutrition*
     *Journal of Fish Diseases*
     *Journal of Veterinary Medicine Series A*
     *Journal of Veterinary Medicine Series B*
     *Journal of Veterinary Pharmacology and Therapeutics*
     *Medical and Veterinary Entomology*
     *Reproduction in Domestic Animals*
     *Veterinary Anaesthesia and Analgesia*

> *Veterinary Dermatology*
> *Veterinary Ophthalmology*

- www.avma.org
  *American Journal of Veterinary Research*
  *Journal of the American Veterinary Medical Association*
- www.j-evs.com
  *Journal of Equine Veterinary Science*
- www.sciencedirect.com
  *Preventive Veterinary Medicine*
  *Research in Veterinary Science*
  *Veterinary Immunology and Immunopathology*
  *Veterinary Journal*
  *Veterinary Microbiology*
  *Veterinary Parasitology*

The following websites also provide access to full-text online versions of journals:

- www.vetrecord.co.uk (figure 3.2) and www.bva.co.uk – provides access to the *Veterinary Record*. Membership of the BVA, or a subscription is required
- www.ingenta.com – provides access to a number of journals on a commercial basis
- www.freemedicaljournals.com – provides free access to a number of medical journals
- highwire.stanford.edu/lists/freeart.dtl – another website providing free access to scientific journals.

Generally the only problem with online journals is that they often don't go back far enough. However, much of the information in the older papers will have

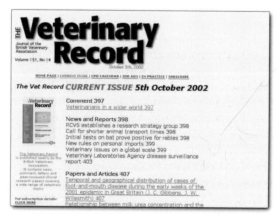

**Fig. 3.2**   An example screen from the *Veterinary Record* website

made its way into the textbooks, and so the online journal remains an excellent, and extremely useful, source for the more recent developments.

### 3.4.2 Textbooks and other review type publications

Most of us consider the use of textbooks, review articles (such as those in continuing professional development (CPD) journals), attendance at CPD lectures, and so on, to be important background knowledge sources. We rely on the specialists and academics to keep up to date with the scientific literature, to combine this with their clinical experience, and then to provide a consensus view for us to apply to our practice.

On the whole the advantages and disadvantages of these sources of information are self-evident. Textbooks are convenient but may be out of date in parts, even on the day of publication. Textbooks are much more digestible than the primary literature but they often represent one person's view of that literature. There are good books and bad books but unfortunately few ways to tell them apart. They remain, and will continue to be, an important secondary information resource. Indeed, there is a considerable, almost palpable, pleasure in owning and using a well-written high-quality textbook that will never be diminished by technological developments, however useful or convenient.

Textbooks can be the source of disinformation. In the 1970s some case reports on a fatal colitis in horses resulting from high doses of oxytetracycline were published. Textbooks published in the 1980s cautioned against the use of this drug in horses as a result of this in spite of the identification for the potential of any broad-spectrum antibiotic to cause the condition. Examination of textbooks suggests that some authors merely paraphrased the information from earlier texts, rather than seriously review the primary data, leading to the possible under-use of a very useful antibiotic in this species.

### 3.4.3 Personal experience and background knowledge

However subjective personal experience might be, it plays an important role in the way we practise veterinary medicine. As the practitioner on the ground we are our own best source of information about local prevalence of disease, or the frequency of post-operative complications following surgery we perform. This information will be flawed due to its subjective nature, because we are not always effective appraisers of our own performance, and are likely to fail to notice common events or give undue prominence to unusual events. A sound basic training in the fundamental biological disciplines enables us to extrapolate information between species and to make rational initial treatment decisions when faced with novel situations.

### 3.4.4  Colleagues

As new graduates we rely heavily on the advice of colleagues until our experience provides the confidence we need to successfully apply the knowledge gained during our veterinary training. New graduates are notorious for a tendency to diagnose rare and unusual conditions while their more experienced colleagues have acquired a better understanding of the relative prevalence of various conditions.

As our clinical skills develop we continue to receive help from more experienced or specialised colleagues seeking information from certificate holders or diplomates. Experts who stay current on the latest evidence from their field may be able to quickly point us at the most relevant literature. We can help our colleagues and ourselves by asking specific questions that are not easily answered from other sources. The use of email and access to colleagues through discussion groups such as the British Small Animal Veterinary Association (BSAVA) website or the Veterinary Information Network (VIN, see below) has made such communication extremely easy and provides an excellent information source for the isolated clinician.

The information gleaned from colleagues, however experienced or specialised, will be subjective and some care must be taken to avoid the propagation of dogma or opinion as evidence.

### 3.4.5  Practice records

The majority of veterinary practices now use some form of computerised record keeping. These systems are normally primarily designed to run the business efficiently rather than to provide epidemiological data. However, it is possible through the use of methodical and consistent coding to use any system to provide practice-specific information on the incidence of disease, post-operative complications, survival rates and the like. This information is often of great value as it is uniquely specific for the local population seen by your practice. This data helps in the interpretation of information obtained from other populations, which either share the characteristics of the local population, or are known to be different in some aspect.

## 3.5  The Internet

The Internet represents a rapidly developing source of primary, secondary and tertiary information that is available both to practitioners and our clients. There is a massive amount of high quality material and an equally massive amount of garbage. Our clients may latch on to either type of information and we need to use our knowledge and skills to either correct our client's misinformed knowledge, or justify our decisions in the face of a well-informed, highly educated client. Newly qualifying graduates have little problem in identifying the Internet as a useful tool for their information needs. For those of us who did not spend our formative years taking computerisation for granted it may be more difficult to see the advantages beyond being able to buy cinema tickets or look up train times.

While on the one hand anyone with a half-baked notion about the curative properties of an untested treatment can post information on the Internet, on the other hand responsible agencies can use it to provide a repository for useful information with a minimal cost to themselves and to those accessing the information. A good example of the latter is the British National Formulary (http://bnf.vhn.net). As new data is added it immediately becomes available to those who need it, and should errors or conflicting information arise, mis-information can be corrected instantly.

So how can we find the useful and not be overwhelmed by the useless? The answer to this is through educating ourselves, and through practice. The main library at the University of Cambridge shelves the books according to size (this is slightly less stupid than it seems and is done to optimise storage capacity). It doesn't render the library unusable but you do need to know how the catalogue works in order to find the book you need. With the Internet you need to know how to use a 'search engine' which is the Internet's equivalent of a catalogue. At the time of writing the author tends to use one called Google (www.google.co.uk or www.google.com) but there are many others available.

The search engine is a website on the Internet that tries to find other websites on the Internet that have the information you require. As a client I might be told that the tumour removed from my dog was a haemangiopericytoma. In Google when I type in 'haemangiopericytoma' it returns with a list of some 250 sites that contain information about this condition both human and veterinary. If I type in the word 'dog' along with 'haemangiopericytoma' I get some 40 results, and if I restrict the findings to UK sites (an option in google.co.uk, which also incidentally recognises that you may also wish to search using the American spelling) I end up with just five (mostly from other owners also looking for information). As a veterinary surgeon giving a talk or preparing a handout I might be interested in some pictures that the search threw up at the Bristol Biomed Image Archive (www.brisbio.ac.uk/ROADS/subject-listing/hemangiopericytoma.html). So with this simple example two important aspects about the Internet have been demonstrated. Firstly there is some useful information out there, and secondly that the Internet is a powerful tool to help the formation or development of community (i.e. enable owners with an interest in a particular disease to communicate). This bringing together of people with a mutual interest is of particular use to veterinary practitioners as we are geographically diverse and have considerable information needs.

This book is not intended to provide general guidance on Internet use, or to provide an exhaustive list of veterinary resources. In general, Internet search strategies work best when the user knows that the information is there (or is highly likely to be there) but doesn't know exactly where. Indeed, a good way of testing the quality of a search engine is to attempt to find a location you already know, and it also provides excellent practice on getting the best out of a search engine.

An excellent tutorial for veterinary Internet use has been made available by the people who produce VetGate (see below). This tutorial can be accessed from the VetGate front page or at: www.vts.rdn.ac.uk/tutorial/vet (figure 3.3).

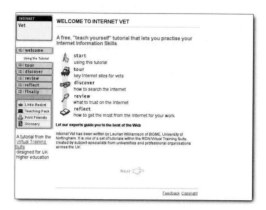

**Fig. 3.3**   An illustration of the veterinary Internet tutorial available via the VetGate website

## 3.6   Veterinary information resources on the Internet

One advantage of the Internet over more traditional print media or CD-ROMs is that it can be constantly updated to include new material. However, the custodians of websites may not be as assiduous as they might be when it comes to updating the information on their websites. Even when using veterinary sites, users should take care to ensure the information presented is reliable and current. The sections below do not represent an exhaustive list and are placed in alphabetical order.

### 3.6.1   CABdirect (www.cabdirect.org)

The CAB International abstract service provides access to an agriculture-based scientific literature abstracts service similar to Medline (see below). It is subscription based, but provides more comprehensive veterinary coverage than Medline. At the time of writing the service could be used for a short period without charge and so readers should be able to evaluate its suitability to their own needs.

### 3.6.2   Consultant (www.vet.cornell.edu/consultant/consult.asp)

Consultant is a diagnostic support system written by Dr Maurice E. White at Cornell University and is available on their website. It is used to suggest possible diagnoses or causes for clinical signs and symptoms, and to provide a brief synopsis of the diagnosis/cause including a general description, the species affected, the signs associated with it, and a list of recent literature references. It uses a database containing approximately 500 signs or symptoms, about 7000 diagnoses/causes, and about 18 000 literature references including over 3000 web references. It can be used to provide possible diagnoses when provided with case-specific information or it can be used to look up the information about a disease. A short, up-to-date list of citations is provided for each disease, which can provide a convenient source of recent papers on a particular condition. The clinical diagnostic support system available on Consultant is described in more detail in Chapter 8.

### 3.6.3   Inno-vet (www.inno-vet.com)

This is an Internet site containing a variety of veterinary information maintained by Dr Ray Markus in the United States. It is noteworthy because it has listings of some veterinary journals not covered in Medline (see below).

### 3.6.4   International Veterinary Information Service (www.ivis.org)

This website, produced by the International Veterinary Information Service, provides access to a number of textbook type documents and abstracts (figure 3.4). IVIS is a not-for-profit organisation, founded in 1998 by veterinary

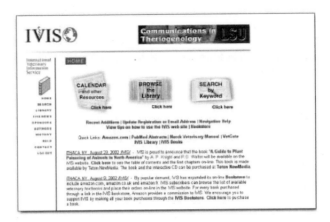

**Fig. 3.4**   The front page of the IVIS website

academic faculty from veterinary colleges and veterinary research institutes in North America, Mexico and Europe. The site requires registration but appears to be funded by sponsorship and limited banner-type advertising. It contains a useful facility for viewing veterinary abstracts on Pubmed (see below), using a number of filters targeting specific veterinary journals and as such provides a useful abstract browsing tool. A number of the IVIS 'books' are listed as 'in preparation', which can be a little frustrating for users.

### 3.6.5   Medline/Pubmed (www.pubmed.org)

Medline is the electronic library of the United States National Library of Medicine. It contains over 10 million citations and is generally considered to be the definitive source of medical evidence. Among the thousands of journals for which it has abstracts are over one hundred veterinary titles (including *The Veterinary Record, Research in Veterinary Science, Vet Clinics of North America*, and many others). Medline is available free of charge through the Pubmed website. Pubmed provides a powerful tool for locating the relevant primary veterinary literature, which together with the RCVS library ensures that any practitioner should be able to find and read any papers they need.

Although searching strategies will be looked at in more detail in the next chapter a quick overview of Pubmed is probably best illustrated by the example below.

A veterinary surgeon has removed a well-circumscribed soft tissue mass from the distal limb of a 7-year-old Labrador Retriever. It is July 2002 and she has just received the histology report which reports the tumour as a haemangiopericytoma. Having achieved a diagnosis she now wishes to be able to advise the client on prognosis. From her personal experience and background knowledge she knows these neoplasms to be malignant but with little tendency to metastasise. What can the literature tell her?

On entering the Pubmed website (figure 3.5) she types hemangiopericytoma (using the American spelling) in the search box and presses the go button. This search yields some 2000 citations because the search is too general, and has included all the human medical citations on the subject. She returns to the search box and adds the word dog. When more than one expression is typed in the search box Pubmed searches Medline for abstracts of papers which contain all the words (i.e. haemagiopericytoma and dog in the same paper). This reduces the yield to a more manageable 40. A quick glance at the titles indicates that relevant papers have been found. It would be no great effort to scan through these citations for those containing information about prognosis but she then decides to add the word prognosis to the searching criteria which narrows the list down to four abstracts (figure 3.6). At the top of the list is a recent paper which is clearly of interest and so she goes on to read the abstract by clicking on the authors' names (figure 3.7). The basic information required is present in the abstract (23 dogs were

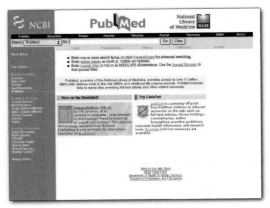

**Fig. 3.5**   The front page of the Pubmed website providing access to the Medline database of scientific papers

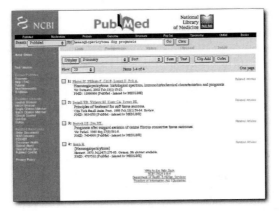

**Fig. 3.6**   The results of a search for papers on the prognosis of canine haemagiopericytoma using Pubmed

followed up for 2 years of which six had a recurrence or metastases). However, she needs access to the full paper in order to make a judgement about the quality of the study and to get the full information. As a recent paper the full text is likely to be available via the Internet. As a member of the RCVS she goes to the college's library website and searches for the journal title in the periodicals section (figure 3.8). She learns that the journal is available to members via the publisher's website. Using the username and password she obtained from the library she locates the journal (figure 3.9) and subsequently the paper itself (figure 3.10). While she could read the paper on screen she prefers to read the printed copy and so gets a copy of the paper in PDF form and prints it from Adobe Acrobat Reader software. The paper itself contains a brief review of the literature in its discussion and these citations can also be pursued for further primary information.

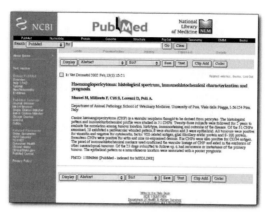

**Fig. 3.7**   A Pubmed screen showing the abstract of a paper from *Veterinary Dermatology* reporting on the prognosis of canine haemangiopericytoma

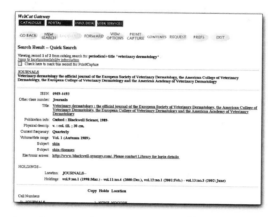

**Fig. 3.8**   Results of a search on the RCVS library website for the journal *Veterinary Dermatology*

Without going into the quality of the data retrieved or the extent of the search performed it is nonetheless clear that primary scientific evidence can be obtained by a typical practitioner in the UK within minutes and at no significant expense. While other searches may not yield the answers to our questions so easily, and we may have to wait for copies of older papers to be sent via the post, the ease and speed at which we have access to the literature will only improve with time.

Listed below are the veterinary journals from which abstracts are available in Medline.

Acta Veterinaria Scandinavica
Acta Veterinaria Scandinavica Supplement
Animal Behaviour

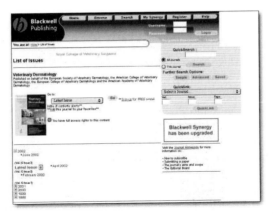

**Fig. 3.9**  The *Veterinary Dermatology* page on the Synergy website

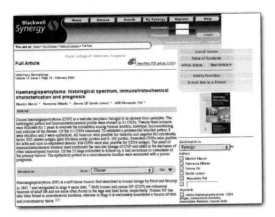

**Fig. 3.10**  The full-text copy of the paper from *Veterinary Dermatology* reporting on the prognosis of canine haemangiopericytoma presented on the Synergy website

Australian Veterinary Journal
Avian Diseases
Clinical Techniques in Small Animal Practice
Domestic Animal Endocrinology
Equine Veterinary Journal
Equine Veterinary Journal Supplement
Journal of the American Animal Hospital Association
Journal of the American Veterinary Medical Association
Journal of Animal Science
Journal of Dairy Science
Journal of Feline Medicine and Surgery
Journal of Parasitology

Journal of Small Animal Practice
Journal of South Africa Veterinary Association
Journal of Veterinary Dentistry
Journal of Veterinary Internal Medicine
Journal of Veterinary Medical Science
Journal of Veterinary Pharmacology and Therapeutics
Journal of Wildlife Diseases
Journal of Zoo and Wildlife Medicine
Laboratory Animal Science
Reproduction in Domestic Animals
Theriogenology
Tierarztliche Praxis
Tropical Animal Health and Production
Veterinary Clinics of North America Equine Practice
Veterinary Clinics of North America Exotic Animal Practice
Veterinary Clinics of North America Food Animal Practice
Veterinary Clinics of North America Small Animal Practice
Veterinary Dermatology
Veterinary Journal (London)
Veterinary Ophthalmology
Veterinary Quarterly
Veterinary Radiology Ultrasound
Veterinary Record
Veterinary Research
Veterinary Surgery

### 3.6.6    The Merck Veterinary Manual (www.merckvetmanual.com)

The *Merck Veterinary Manual* (MVM) is a well-established conventional textbook on general animal health. The MVM is published on a non-profit basis through a cooperative effort between Merck & Co, Inc. and Merial Limited as a service to the veterinary profession. The full text and illustrations are available on CD-ROM and via the website (figure 3.11). A flexible searching tool is provided on the website in addition to the conventional book's contents structure.

### 3.6.7    Montreal Veterinary School (www.medvet.umontreal.ca/biblio/vetjr.html)

The website of Montreal Veterinary School in Canada has an online listing of veterinary journals linking to Pubmed if the journal is indexed by Medline, or the websites of the journals themselves. A number of journals and conference proceedings not included in Medline can be searched using this site.

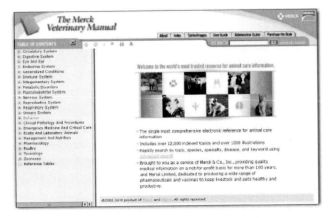

**Fig. 3.11**  An example page from the Merck Veterinary Manual website

### 3.6.8  *NetVet and the Electronic Zoo (www.netvet.wustl.edu)*

This website currently hosted by Washington University is a long-established veterinary site for veterinary surgeons (NetVet) and the public (the Electronic Zoo) established by Dr Ken Boschert (figure 3.12). It may have been moved to the American Veterinary Medical Association site by the time this book goes to press (www.avma.org). This site contains a fairly comprehensive collection of links to other veterinary websites throughout the world. Ken Boschert is also a co-author of *Mosby's Guide to the Internet,* another guide to veterinary sites on the Internet with an accompanying website (www.us.elsevierhealth.com/MERLIN/netvet/).

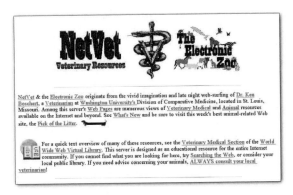

**Fig. 3.12**  The front page of the NetVet website

### 3.6.9   *RCVS (www.rcvs.org.uk) and RCVS library (www.rcvslibrary.org.uk)*

The RCVS website provides useful access to the RCVS library and information
service. The RCVS provides some access to some full-text online versions of
veterinary journals to members of the college (user IDs and passwords can be
requested from the RCVS). With easy public access to abstract databases such as
Medline (see above) one of the greatest obstacles to the practice of EBVM is
getting access to journals. Most practising veterinary surgeons do not have easy
access to comprehensive libraries but the RCVS library through its reprint service and by providing online access goes some way to meet this need. There are
also some useful links to EBM and EBVM sites on the RCVS website.

### 3.6.10   *VetGate (www.vetgate.ac.uk)*

This is a website providing access to other Internet resources in animal health,
veterinary medicine and related topics (figure 3.13). It has been built by a
consortium led by the University of Nottingham Greenfield Medical Library
including the RCVS Library and Information Service and the Royal Veterinary
College. It provides some of the functionality of a general Internet search engine
but is restricted to veterinary information.

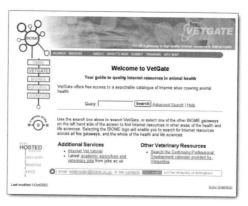

**Fig. 3.13**   The front page of the VetGate website

### 3.6.11   *VIN (www.vin.com)*

Veterinary Information Network (figure 3.14) is a commercially run site (i.e.
users pay a subscription) which is restricted to qualified vets. At the time of
writing new users can take advantage of a free trial. The site is based in the US
with an associated North American slant to the material. Abstracts from a wide
variety of veterinary journals can be accessed through the site together with a

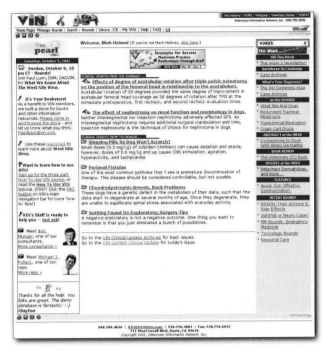

**Fig. 3.14**   The front page of the Veterinary Information Network website

wealth of other educational material. One of the site's great strengths is the collection of discussion forums where vets post questions. These questions are normally answered by a board certified clinician employed by VIN and may be discussed by other participating vets.

### 3.6.12   Wildlife Information Network (www.wildlifeinformation.org)

The Wildlife Information Network (WIN), produces information on the health and management of wild animals and their habitats for veterinary surgeons and other wildlife professionals. They distribute this information through their website and via a CD-ROM. They are a charitable organisation and charge a subscription for access. Further details can be found on their website.

## 3.7   Other computer-based information resources

A number of databases and other computerised resources containing veterinary information exist which are not available on the Internet. Most of these are currently available on CD-ROMs although it seems likely that some will be transferred to Internet access in the fullness of time. The list of resources below is not exhaustive but does indicate the range of material available.

### 3.7.1    BSAVA

The British Small Animal Veterinary Association (BSAVA) has long had a good reputation for its congress, courses, journal and books. Over the years they have also produced a number of CD-ROMs. Some of these just contain recordings of talks given at their annual congress while others contain more interactive packages. Their small animal case simulations and their radiology disc merit a mention. Further details can be obtained from their website at www.bsava.com.

### 3.7.2    CLIVE

The acronym CLIVE stands for the Consortium for Learning in Veterinary Education and was formed to help produce and distribute computer aided learning materials among the UK veterinary schools. Under the leadership of Dr Andrew Short, they have produced a large number of CD-ROMs, which are used throughout the world. Although primarily aimed at the undergraduate curriculum, many of the packages produced are available commercially. Details of the packages and more information about CLIVE can be obtained from the CLIVE website, www.clive.ed.ac.uk. Although a member of CLIVE, the Royal Veterinary College also has its own continuing education organisation from which educational CD-ROMs can be obtained. Details can be found on the CPD page of their website, www.rvc.ac.uk.

### 3.7.3    Lifelearn

Lifelearn is another commercial enterprise producing educational material for vets. Their primary market is the North American veterinary practitioner although they also have a UK retail organisation. They originally produced interactive CD-ROMs using the CDi system. They subsequently converted their products for use on Windows PCs. They are well-made educational materials and, like the CLIVE and BSAVA discs, represent a good way of improving background knowledge in the areas covered. Their website address is www.lifelearn.com.

### 3.7.4    Vetstream

Vetstream is the vision of John Grieve, a small animal practitioner who was quick to spot the potential for the use of information technology to provide a medium for accessing veterinary information. It is currently delivered on CD-ROMs, which are provided to veterinary surgeons on a subscription basis. They provide coverage of four species, the dog, cat, horse and rabbit. The CD-ROMs are produced by a large team of writers and editors. They represent an encyclopaedic interactive textbook, containing information in the form of text, pictures, sound and video. The editorial process includes a peer review process, but the content is largely secondary in nature, although extremely comprehensive. There is a very consistent structure to the articles, which enables users to find the information quickly and easily. At the time of writing, there are plans to offer an Internet service. Their website can be found at www.vetstream.co.uk.

## 3.8   Critically appraised topics

As these do not exist in veterinary medicine this section might be regarded as redundant. Critically appraised topics, or CATs, are common in human EBM. They are short summaries of the evidence to a focused clinical question. When someone has already looked for the evidence to answer a question it allows them to store the results of their critical appraisal in such a way that they can be shared or stored for later use. In essence it is a way of sharing the workload of appraisal for commonly asked questions. In the medical world they are to be found on various websites (e.g. www.indigojazz.co.uk/CEBM/cats.asp). They (should) have a relatively short 'shelf life' and so the Internet is a good place to store and share them.

Perhaps the veterinary community could benefit from adopting this strategy?

## Further reading

Boschert, K. and James, H. (1998) *NetVet: Mosby's Guide to the Internet.* Mosby Year Book, New York.

## Review questions

Choose the best single answer for the following questions. Answers on page 204

**1** *Which of the following represents the weakest form of evidence?*

    (a)   A letter in a CPD journal
    (b)   A peer-reviewed article in a journal
    (c)   Drug company literature
    (d)   A recommendation from a colleague.

**2** *On which website can you access full-text from the journal Veterinary Dermatology?*

    (a)   www.blackwell-synergy.com
    (b)   www.avma.com
    (c)   www.j-evs.com
    (d)   www.sciencedirect.com
    (e)   www.ingenta.com

**3** *The Pubmed website provides access to which database?*

    (a)   CAB abstracts
    (b)   Medlar
    (c)   Medline
    (d)   Consultant
    (e)   Vetstream
    (f)   RCVS library catalogue
    (g)   All of the above.

**4** *Which of the following website subscriptions is not available to members of the RCVS?*

    (a)   www.blackwell-synergy.com
    (b)   www.avma.com
    (c)   www.j-evs.com
    (d)   www.sciencedirect.com
    (e)   www.ingenta.com

**5** *What is a CAT?*

    (a)   An animal chased by a DOG
    (b)   A Critically Appraised Topic
    (c)   A summary of the evidence available to answer a particular clinical question
    (d)   All of the above.

# 4

# SEARCHING FOR EVIDENCE

The objective of this chapter is to introduce the processes by which evidence can be found. The chapter will concentrate on searching computer-based resources via the Internet with particular emphasis on how Medline can be interrogated using Pubmed in order to search the veterinary literature.

After reading this chapter the reader should be able to:

- Use general library resources such as the RCVS and Consultant websites to find secondary sources of evidence
- Understand the principles of using Boolean logic when searching Pubmed for primary scientific papers
- Broaden or narrow searches to improve sensitivity and specificity of searches on Pubmed
- Find abstracts on therapy, diagnosis, aetiology, and prognosis

## 4.1   Introduction

Every practitioner will have a collection of student notes, journals, textbooks, course notes and so on, with which they will be familiar. Some practices are within easy reach of a good university library from which they may also be able to access books and journals. These are all good sources of primary and secondary scientific information and readers will probably need no additional guidance on how to use them. This chapter will concentrate on Internet-based resources with which readers may not be familiar, but to which all readers are likely to have ready access, no matter where they are located.

## 4.2   RCVS library

As mentioned in the previous chapter, the Royal College of Veterinary Surgeons (RCVS) library catalogue is a much under-used resource. In recent years considerable efforts have been made to ensure that the catalogue is easily usable online. Book loans can be requested from the website as well as journal papers. Recent acquisitions can be viewed separately which provides a useful way of looking out for new publications. Registration for electronic use of the library can be performed by sending an email to the librarian (details are given on their website). In the previous chapter, access to full-text online journals available to members of the RCVS is described. An example from the online catalogue is shown in figure 4.1.

## 4.3   Other online book catalogues

There are a number of useful websites that can be used to search for veterinary publications. The online bookseller Amazon (www.amazon.co.uk or

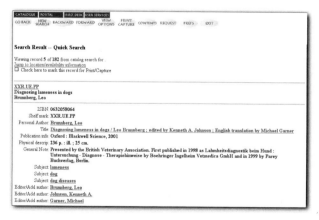

**Fig. 4.1**   An example of a book catalogue record from the RCVS library website

www.amazon.com) provides a comprehensive catalogue of books in print which includes veterinary titles. Although the marketing efforts of the publishers rarely fail to keep us informed we tend not to keep the unsolicited mail handy when we finally get round to looking for a better book on therapeutics. A quick search using a few key words that you might expect to find in the title of a desired text will often turn up a suitable book.

Other bookshop websites that may be useful include Blackwells (www.bookshop.blackwell.co.uk), Bookpoint (www.zc74.dial.pipex.com), Cairns (www.vet-books.co.uk), Houghtons (www.houghtonbooks.com), and Profbooks.com (www.profbooks.com).

University library catalogues such as that of the University of Cambridge are also a useful way of locating the details of a book that may be worth reading.

## 4.4   Consultant

Cornell University's Consultant website provides a useful way of obtaining references to primary and secondary literature sources. From the home page individual diseases or signs of disease may be looked up providing a list of additional printed sources of information (an example is shown in figure 4.2). Many of these references are recent overviews of the subject from educational journals as well as citations from the primary scientific literature.

## 4.5   Searching strategies: simple Boolean logic

Any reader who has spent time using the Internet will have been frustrated by the difficulty in finding the information for which they are searching. When

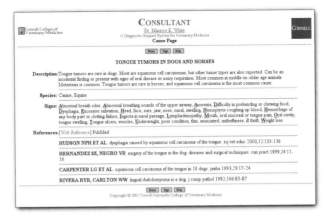

**Fig. 4.2**   An example of the information available from the Consultant website

searching the Internet we are either overwhelmed by the amount of data, 99% of which seems to be either irrelevant or useless, or we fail to find the specific thing we require (we know it must be there, but cannot locate it). We can never avoid this entirely but we can improve our success rate by learning how to search effectively and develop strategies to improve our efficiency.

The first step in this process is to understand a little Boolean logic. This is nothing difficult; it is something we use every day. When I go to the bookshop to choose a novel to take on holiday, in order to reach this decision I probably have a few authors I like to read but don't want one I've read before. For example, I might like Ian Rankin's novels and Agatha Christie's Poirot novels (but not her Miss Marple books). In order to choose a book I intuitively perform some Boolean logic. The book I choose is written either by Ian Rankin or an Agatha Christie which features Poirot, but not one I've read before. In logical terms, this can be described as follows:

((Author is Ian Rankin) OR (Author is Agatha Christie AND Hero is Poirot)) AND previously unread

The Boolean operators OR and AND are used to include or exclude items in our search, and the brackets are used to separate elements in the search. Sometimes an easier way of excluding items is to use the 'NOT' operator. Thus to exclude the previously read books we could replace 'AND previously unread' with 'NOT previously read'. The brackets are used just to make it clear how (in what order) the operations should be performed.

## 4.6  Using Pubmed

In order to retrieve papers from Pubmed we type one or more key words in the search box to direct the search. Pubmed also permits the use of logical operators to refine the search. If several key words are typed into the search box Pubmed performs a logical AND.

So if we were searching for evidence to help in the selection of a suitable non-steroidal anti-inflammatory to use for post-surgical analgesia we could type: 'dog NSAID surgery' into the box which would retrieve abstracts each of which is indexed using the word 'dog' and the word 'NSAID' and the word 'surgery' (called MeSH terms described briefly below). We could have typed the query as 'dog AND NSAID AND surgery'.

At the time of writing, this search produced 166 abstracts, which is more than I would want to read at one sitting. It is also evident that many of these papers are not particularly relevant, many of them reporting on esoteric non-clinical research. Clearly the papers we are more interested in are those reporting the results of clinical trials. We need to narrow down the search.

The following query will focus in on the papers of interest:

Dog NSAID surgery 'randomised controlled trial' [PTYP] OR 'drug therapy' [SH] OR 'therapeutic use' [SH:NOEXP] OR 'random*' [WORD]

Suddenly everything looks a lot more complicated, but with a little deconstruction it isn't so difficult to understand.

The previous search terms 'dog NSAID surgery' are included at the beginning as before. Pubmed will AND these with the following part of the query.

To understand the additional part of the query it is worth considering the additional information that is stored with the abstract which is added by the National Library of Medicine (NLM), to help their retrieval. Each abstract is indexed using one or more subject headings. NLM's Medical Subject Headings (MeSH) are a predefined set of biomedical terms used to describe the subject of each abstract. MeSH contains more than 19 000 terms and is updated annually to reflect changes in medical terminology. MeSH terms are arranged hierarchically by subject categories with more specific terms arranged beneath broader terms. MeSH headings automatically include the more specific subheading terms under the term in a search unless they are specifically excluded. The abbreviations SH for MeSH subheading, and MH for MeSH term will be encountered frequently in descriptions or accounts of Medline searching. Additional data stored includes the publication type such as journal article, review, editorial, or randomised controlled trial.

Returning to the example, we see that the remaining part of the query narrows the search by using the other search terms (listed below) and looks for any abstract with one or more of the following (performs a logical OR):

'randomised controlled trial' [PTYP]
'drug therapy' [SH]
'therapeutic use' [SH:NOEXP]
'random*' [WORD]

What do these search terms find?

The first one, 'randomised controlled trial' [PTYP] looks for the term 'randomised controlled trial' as the publication type.

The second one looks for abstracts having a 'drug therapy' entry in their MeSH subheading.

The third one looks for 'therapeutic use' in the MeSH subheading (but not for any expanded terms included which are listed as further subheadings of this term).

The final item looks for the word 'random' or any word beginning with these letters in the body text or title of the abstract. (The asterisk is a wildcard character representing zero or more unspecified characters at the end of a word; a question mark can be used to match a single unknown character within a word.) This will pick up the words random, randomised, and randomising.

When this search is performed it reduces the yield by half, most being clinically relevant but many papers are not reporting the results of well-controlled clinical trials. To use an epidemiological term, we have high sensitivity (we found all the true positives) but we have a lower specificity (we didn't exclude all the true negatives).

As we are primarily interested in clinical trials which are single or double blinded, or use placebos we could use the following alternative command to narrow down the search:

(dog nsaid surgery) AND (((single [WORD] OR double [WORD]) AND blind* [WORD]) OR placebo [WORD])

This yields only one-tenth of the abstracts originally located, all of which describe the results of well-controlled clinical trials.

## 4.7    Sensitivity and specificity

In just the same way that the cut-off point that we use in any diagnostic test needs to be adjusted to avoid too many false positives in a common disease, or avoid too many false negatives in a rare disease, we may need to adjust our search strategies depending on the depth of the literature. Haynes *et al.* (1994) describe a number of strategies designed to increase either the sensitivity or specificity of searches.

In general it pays to start with a more sensitive search. Pubmed provides the facility to further search within the results which helps to locate the abstracts of interest without sacrificing sensitivity. Greater familiarity with the MeSH system can also help to choose the most appropriate terminology. A MeSH browser is available on Pubmed for this purpose (illustrated in figure 4.3).

To increase sensitivity the following may help:

- Expand the search using broader MeSH terms
- Use the [WORD] option to search for text within the body of the abstract
- Use the * or ? characters to find variants of words
- Use the Boolean OR to ensure alternatives for the terms you are after.

To increase the specificity the following may help:

- Use more narrow MeSH terms (with the [SH:NOEXP] option if appropriate)
- Use the Boolean AND to narrow the scope of the search
- Limit the search by publication type, year of publication and so on.

## 4.8    Special veterinary considerations

There are occasions when just using the species name alone provides a suffi-cient filter to retrieve veterinary abstracts. However, the use of the enzyme

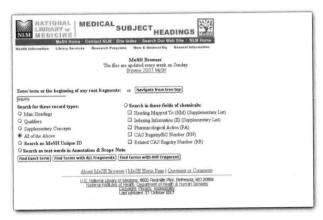

**Fig. 4.3**   The front page of the Medical Subject Headings browser available via the Pubmed website

horseradish peroxidase in ELISA tests means that using the word horse during a search can yield some unlikely results. Similarly the use of cats and dogs as experimental animals may also provide an excessive number of abstracts. While these searches can provide useful evidence serendipitously, the addition of the word 'veterinary' to searches will normally solve the problem.

## 4.9   Searching for the answers to questions about therapy

For a veterinary clinical query on therapy with an emphasis on achieving high sensitivity the following query can be used. If more than one species is of interest these can be 'OR'ed together. The MeSH system includes concepts such as ruminants, Linaean nomenclature etc.

> *Your query* AND *species* AND ('randomised controlled trial' [PTYP] OR 'drug therapy' [SH] OR 'therapeutic use' [SH:NOEXP] OR 'random*' [WORD])

A more specific query on veterinary therapy can be made using the following text.

> *Your query* AND *species* AND veterinary AND ((double [WORD] OR single [WORD]) AND blind* [WORD]) OR placebo [WORD]

Although in a perfect world it would be desirable to limit this search to double-blinded trials it is reasonable to believe that single-blinded veterinary trials are less affected by placebo effect than similar human studies.

## 4.10   Searching for the answers to questions about diagnosis

For a search emphasising sensitivity the following search may be used which looks for MeSH term 'sensitivity and specificity', those two words within the abstract, or the MeSH terms 'diagnosis' or 'diagnostic use'.

> *Your query* AND *species* AND ('sensitivity and specificity' [MESH] OR 'sensitivity' [WORD] OR 'diagnosis' [SH] OR 'diagnostic use' [SH] OR 'specificity' [WORD])

For a more specific search the following query can be used.

> *Your query* AND *species* AND veterinary AND ('sensitivity and specificity' [MESH] OR ('predictive' [WORD] AND 'value*' [WORD]))

This search looks for papers with the MeSH term 'sensitivity and specificity' or with a mention of predictive value(s) within the text.

## 4.11   Searching for the answers to questions about aetiology

For a search on the aetiology of a veterinary disease emphasising sensitivity the following query could be used. This searches for the MeSH terms 'risk', 'cohort studies' and 'case–control studies', together with these words together with 'risk' within the text of the abstract.

> *Your query* AND *species* AND ('cohort studies' [MESH] OR 'risk' [MESH] OR ('odds' [WORD] AND 'ratio*' [WORD]) OR ('relative' [WORD] AND 'risk' [WORD]) OR 'case' control*' [WORD] OR case–control studies [MESH])

A more specific query about aetiology can be made with the following text.

> *Your query* AND *species* AND veterinary AND ('case–control studies' [MH:NOEXP] OR 'cohort studies' [MH:NOEXP])

This search looks only for abstracts indexed with the MeSH headings 'veterinary', 'case–control studies' or 'cohort studies'.

## 4.12   Searching for the answers to questions about prognosis

For a search on the prognosis of a disease the following query can be used. The MeSH terms 'incidence', 'follow-up studies' or 'mortality' will find an abstract together with the words 'prognosis' and 'predict' in the text.

> *Your query* AND *species* AND ('incidence' [MESH] OR 'mortality' [MESH] OR 'follow-up studies' [MESH] OR 'mortality' [SH] OR prognos* [WORD] OR predict* [WORD] OR course [WORD])

A more specific search yielding veterinary papers indexed with the MeSH terms 'prognosis' and 'survival analysis' (without subheading expansion) is performed with the following query.

> *Your query* AND *species* AND veterinary AND (prognosis [MH:NOEXP] OR 'survival analysis' [MH:NOEXP])

## 4.13 Using the 'Clinical Queries' option in Pubmed

Searches very similar to those described above can be performed with a minimum of extra typing by using the 'Clinical Queries' option in Pubmed (see figure 4.4). The filters used are listed in table 4.1 together with the sensitivities and specificities of these searches when used to perform medical queries.

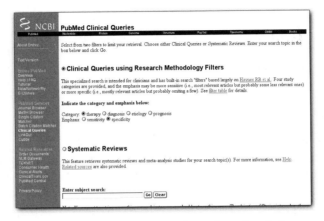

**Fig. 4.4** The clinical queries page from the Pubmed website

## 4.14 Depth of the veterinary scientific literature

Although we may feel like a 'Cinderella' profession when it comes to resources available for the practice of EBVM, as compared with the medical profession, the primary veterinary literature does exist. Table 4.2 summarises the number of papers for each of the main veterinary species contained in the Medline database. Details of papers dating from 1966 to the present are available, although abstracts may not be available for the older papers. Much of it will be of little use to an individual's veterinary practice, but in that total of around 250 000 papers that appear to have clinical relevance to clinical veterinary medicine, are a few that could make an enormous difference to patients, their owners, and your own satisfaction resulting from doing a better job.

**Table 4.1** Search filters used by Pubmed for Clinical Query searches.

| Question | Sensitivity/ specificity* | Pubmed search filter |
|---|---|---|
| *Therapy* | | |
| Sensitive | 99%/74% | 'randomised controlled trial' [PTYP] OR 'drug therapy' [SH] OR 'therapeutic use' [SH:NOEXP] OR 'random*' [WORD] |
| Specific | 57%/97% | (double [WORD] AND blind* [WORD]) OR placebo [WORD] |
| *Diagnosis* | | |
| Sensitive | 92%/73% | 'sensitivity and specificity' [MESH] OR 'sensitivity' [WORD] OR 'diagnosis' [SH] OR 'diagnostic use' [SH] OR 'specificity' [WORD] |
| Specific | 55%/98% | 'sensitivity and specificity' [MESH] OR ('predictive' [WORD] AND 'value*' [WORD]) |
| *Aetiology* | | |
| Sensitive | 82%/70% | 'cohort studies' [MESH] OR 'risk' [MESH] OR ('odds' [WORD] AND 'ratio*' [WORD]) OR ('relative' [WORD] AND 'risk' [WORD]) OR 'case' control* [WORD] OR case-control studies [MESH] |
| Specific | 40%/98% | 'case-control studies' [MH:NOEXP] OR 'cohort studies' [MH:NOEXP] |
| *Prognosis* | | |
| Sensitive | 92%/73% | 'incidence' [MESH] OR 'mortality' [MESH] OR 'follow-up studies' [MESH] OR 'mortality' [SH] OR prognos* [WORD] OR predict* [WORD] OR course [WORD] |
| Specific | 49%/97% | prognosis [MH:NOEXP] OR 'survival analysis' [MH:NOEXP] |

Sensitivity and specificity from Haynes *et al.* (1994).

**Table 4.2** Number of abstracts available in July 2002 from Clinical Query searches on Pubmed for each of the main veterinary species.

| Question | Dog | Cat | Horse | Cow | Sheep |
|---|---|---|---|---|---|
| *Therapy* | | | | | |
| Sensitive | 22 938 | 6725 | 3601 | 12 157 | 5987 |
| Specific | 805 | 237 | 181 | 462 | 203 |
| *Diagnosis* | | | | | |
| Sensitive | 53 833 | 22 604 | 11 769 | 40 417 | 19 161 |
| Specific | 1246 | 539 | 458 | 2085 | 696 |
| *Aetiology* | | | | | |
| Sensitive | 4364 | 1892 | 1280 | 2738 | 965 |
| Specific | 267 | 197 | 136 | 363 | 106 |
| *Prognosis* | | | | | |
| Sensitive | 11 134 | 5264 | 2496 | 9206 | 3978 |
| Specific | 1090 | 396 | 341 | 239 | 139 |

## 4.15 Developing searching skills

While the breadth and depth of the veterinary literature may not always provide a source of primary scientific evidence for answering a question about a particular clinical case, it is undeniable that as each year passes the literature expands and improves. Just as our clinical skills improve with time and experience, our searching skills also improve with use. Being able to find primary scientific papers, which provide the evidence on which we base our decisions, is clearly central to the practice of EBVM. It cannot be denied that it can be frustrating while on the steep part of the learning curve but it is also immensely rewarding to be able to find, appraise and apply newly acquired information in the treatment of a patient. It is also rewarding to share this information with colleagues and be able to use our access to expert colleagues to help us interpret this information, rather than just rely on the experts to pass on this knowledge second-hand.

## References and websites

Haynes, R.B., Wilczynski, N., McKibbon, K.A., Walker, C.J. and Sinclair, J.C. (1994) Developing optimal search strategies for detecting clinically sound studies in MEDLINE. *J Am Med Inform Assoc* **1** (6), 447–58.

Amazon: www.amazon.co.uk (or www.amazon.com for the US site, which isn't identical)

Consultant: www.vet.cornell.edu/consultant/Consult.asp

MeSH Browser: www.nlm.nih.gov/mesh/meshhome.html

Pubmed Clinical Queries: www.ncbi.nlm.nih.gov:80/entrez/query/static/clinical.html

Pubmed help and tutorial are available from the Pubmed home page

Pubmed: www.ncbi.nlm.nih.gov/entrez/query.fcgi

RCVS library: www.rcvslibrary.org.uk/

University of Cambridge library catalogue: www.lib.cam.ac.uk/public_info.html

## Review questions

Choose the best single answer for the following questions. Answers on page 204

**1** *What does the Pubmed search 'therapeutic use [SH:NOEXP]' do?*

(a)  Search for papers containing the words therapeutic use
(b)  Search for papers containing the words therapeutic use in the title
(c)  Search for papers containing stored under the subject heading therapeutic use, or any other keyword with a meaning that is a subset of therapeutic use
(d)  Search for papers containing stored under the subject heading therapeutic use, without searching for papers stored under any other keyword.

**2** *If you were performing a sensitive search, how many papers would you expect to find compared to a more specific search?*

(a)  More
(b)  Less
(c)  The same.

**3** *On Pubmed, if you wanted to find all words beginning with the letters 'haemo' what text would you need to type?*

(a)  Ha?mo
(b)  Hemo?
(c)  He*mo
(d)  Haemo*
(e)  Haemo???????

**4** *What are the four predefined categories of paper that can be searched for using the clinical queries facility on Pubmed?*

(a)  Therapy, diagnosis, aetiology, and prognosis
(b)  Therapy (sensitive), therapy (specific), diagnosis (sensitive), diagnosis (specific)
(c)  Human, murine, feline and canine.

**5** *What are the main Boolean logic operators used in database searching?*

(a)  AND, OR and NOT
(b)  EOR, OR, and NOR
(c)  IF, AND and BUT
(d)  All of the above.

# 5

# RESEARCH
# STUDIES

The aim of this chapter is to enable the reader to understand the strengths and weaknesses of the different types of studies and thereby be able to identify the studies of greatest relevance to their own questions.

After reading this chapter the reader should:

- Understand the structures of different types of studies
- Understand the advantages and disadvantages of each design
- Understand the evidence hierarchy and how this relates to the power of a study
- Be able to identify the type of study required to answer a clinical question.

## 5.1    Hierarchy of evidence and experimental design

The hierarchy of evidence is a broad categorisation of sources highlighting those that are the most likely to produce the best evidence. In most clinical situations the value of evidence is directly proportional to the statistical power of the study. The power of the study indicates the ability of the study to demonstrate a difference. The power of a study is dependent on the size of the study population, the magnitude of the effect of the intervention, and the natural variation in the parameters being measured.

The study design can reduce the natural variation of the measured parameters and increase the power of the study. This allows the construction of a hierarchy of evidence based on the power of different study designs to answer specific research questions. The object of the evidence hierarchy is to concentrate the effort on the sources most likely to yield the greatest rewards.

The greatest statistical certainty comes from well-conducted meta-analyses that incorporate a number of randomised controlled experimental studies. Because of the large number of participants the results are more reflective of the population as a whole. The randomised controlled trial (RCT) will always have the greatest power when compared to other data collection designs but it may not be appropriate to answer questions about causation where cohorts or case–control studies are more appropriate. RCTs are the design of choice for evidence regarding treatments. Trial designs further down the pyramid produce results that are less transferable to other populations but may be more applicable to certain types of patient. An example of an evidence pyramid for published sources of information is shown in figure 5.1. The least clinically relevant

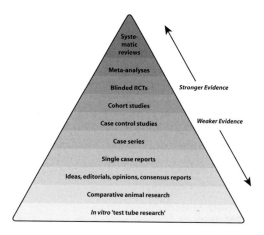

**Fig. 5.1**    The hierarchy of published evidence illustrated as a pyramid of evidence

sources are at the bottom of the pyramid and the most clinically relevant sources are shown at the top of the pyramid.

Hierarchies are guides to the power of the designs, but the quality of the individual studies needs to be critically appraised. There is overlap between the different levels in the hierarchy since a well-designed cohort study may provide better evidence than a poorly designed RCT. The hierarchy does not exclude data from other sources but alerts the clinician to the critical appraisal of the available evidence, or prompts the search for a study to provide better evidence.

When few higher quality sources of evidence are available representing the apex of the pyramid we can work down the hierarchy until sufficient information is obtained. Individual case reports may be extremely helpful in the absence of any other information. Alternatively, when searches yield an excessive numbers of articles, we can concentrate on the better evidence by filtering out the results of studies lower in the hierarchy.

In veterinary medicine we are often faced with a relative paucity of trial data but it is nonetheless important to be conscious of the shortcomings of the few available studies, and note lack of strong evidence in many instances.

## 5.2   Guide to research methods

The following sections are a basic guide to understanding the different types of study designs and how the design can influence the evidence it provides.

Studies can be divided into descriptive studies and explanatory studies.

Descriptive studies are designed to record observations. They do not compare the observations to a control group and therefore no attempt should be made to explain causation or make conclusions about treatment effects. They can be used for formulating hypotheses that can be tested by more appropriate and powerful explanatory designed studies.

Explanatory studies differ from descriptive studies as they compare two groups. The comparison may be between diseased and non-diseased animals with regard to a disease risk factor, or it may be an evaluation of a new treatment where one group is treated with a traditional treatment, while the other group receives the new treatment. The groups are then examined and outcomes compared. There are two main types of explanatory study, experimental and observational. In experimental studies the animals are randomly allocated to different treatment groups. In observational studies the groups are created from the treatments the animals have had or are receiving.

## 5.3   Literature reviews

In general, a good systematic review or a meta-analysis will provide stronger evidence than an individual study.

## 5.3.1   *Systematic reviews*

Ideally, important veterinary questions should be studied more than once by different research teams in different locations. Systematic reviews and meta-analyses can be used to increase the evidence provided by these individual studies (figure 5.2).

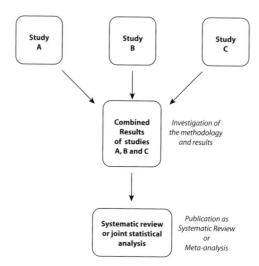

**Fig. 5.2**   A schematic representation of the process of performing systematic reviews and meta-analyses

A systematic review is a comprehensive survey of a topic in which all the primary studies of the highest level of evidence have been systematically identified, appraised and then summarised according to explicit and reproducible methodologies. Reviews are potentially a good source of information for the busy veterinarian. The best reviews should provide unbiased summaries of all the available evidence.

## 5.3.2   *Meta-analyses*

A meta-analysis is a survey in which the designs of all the included studies are similar enough statistically that the results can be combined and analysed as if they were a single study. The studies should include a thorough search of the literature with defined criteria for study inclusion or exclusion.

The results of a meta-analysis are usually presented in a forest plot indicating the odds ratio and the confidence intervals of the individual and combined studies. An example of a forest plot of a meta-analysis is shown in figure 5.3. An odds

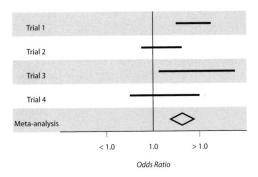

**Fig. 5.3** An illustration of how the results of a meta-analysis are summarised graphically

ratio of 1 indicates no effect. An odds ratio of greater than 1 indicates an improvement and an odds ratio less than 1 indicates a decline.

If all the horizontal lines indicating the 95% confidence intervals of the trial results overlap as they do in figure 5.3, then the results are compatible and there is said to be homogeneity of the results. It is therefore likely that it is justifiable to combine the data from the studies as they give similar results. If they do not overlap, the results show heterogeneity, and this implies that the results are significantly different in some respect, and the results should probably not be pooled. The heterogeneity may be due to differences between the trials in respect of the populations, methodology or operator bias. Sometimes a sensitivity analysis is performed where the methods used and the studies are changed to check for consistency of the results obtained. If the results remain consistent then there is greater confidence in the reliability of the results.

## 5.4 Experimental studies

Experimental studies are those over which the investigator determines the method of selection of the animals studied, and the interventions they receive.

### 5.4.1 Randomised controlled trials

Randomised controlled trials may be experimental laboratory studies or experimental clinical trials.

Experimental laboratory studies use experimental animals and reduce the variables by controlling the environment. The researcher has control over the allocation of animals into the groups being compared and the administration of the treatments to these groups. This method provides the best evidence of cause, or treatment effect. However, the results may lack relevance to the real world.

Experimental clinical trials use privately owned animals and the animals are kept in their normal environment. The disease in the animal is naturally occurring. Animals are usually allocated by the researcher to the treatment groups, but there is little or no direct control over treatment administration. If the protocols are well designed and performed properly, clinical trials provide the best evidence for the outcome that can be expected if the intervention is adopted for use in a population under field conditions.

An RCT has two important features (figure 5.4):

- There are at least two groups: one or more treatment groups, and a control group. The treatment group receives the treatment or intervention under investigation and the control group receives either no treatment or a standard default. The standard default contains all the ingredients at the same concentrations as the treatment but does not contain the active ingredient under investigation. This also acts as a placebo so that the owner does not know if their animal is in the treatment or the control group.
- Patients are randomly assigned to the two groups.

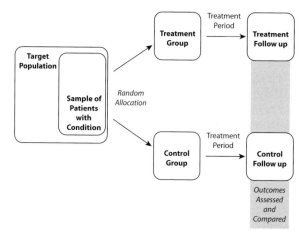

**Fig. 5.4**   A schematic representation of a randomised controlled trial

The two groups are observed in an identical fashion. The groups are followed for a specific length of time at which point the trial ends. Any differences in the trial outcome are attributable to the trial. Double blinding should be used if possible. A trial in which neither the owner/animal, or the veterinary surgeon knows which treatment the animal is receiving is called double blind. This avoids bias and ensures that each group, whether treatment or control, will have an equivalent placebo effect, i.e. an improvement caused by giving the patient/ owner something. The measured outcome therefore relates to the actual treatment not the act of giving a treatment.

The control group allows a comparison to be made between the treatment and a chosen alternative, such as no treatment, or an alternative therapy. This is important as an excellent cure rate without a control may simply reflect the outcome of the natural course of the disease irrespective of the treatment used.

The RCT is the design of choice for answering questions about the effectiveness of different treatments, and a search for evidence from this study design should be a priority when asking questions about therapies.

*Advantages*

- Random allocation reduces the risk of bias and is the most powerful method of eliminating known and unknown confounding variables
- It is the most powerful study design for data collection
- It increases the probability that the differences between the groups can be attributed to the treatment.

*Disadvantages*

- Sometimes it is unethical to allow for an untreated control group due to the severity of the effects of withholding an effective treatment
- These studies are expensive to conduct and relatively rare in veterinary medicine.

### 5.4.2   Cross-over designs

A sample population is randomly assigned to one of two treatment groups and followed over time to see if they develop the outcome of interest. After a period of time during which the outcome would have been expected to occur they are switched to the other treatment sometimes with a washout period in between (figure 5.5). They are then monitored for a further period and the outcomes during this period noted.

*Advantage*

Because the subjects act as their own control the number of animals can be reduced compared to an RCT.

*Disadvantage*

Treatments with persistent actions confound the results.

## 5.5   Observational studies

Like experimental studies observational studies are explanatory in nature, with a comparison between two groups. However, unlike experimental studies the

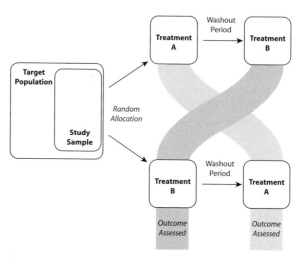

**Fig. 5.5**   A schematic representation of a cross-over study

allocation of the study animals to the groups being compared is not under the control of the researcher although matching of the individuals selected for the study is. The power of the study is therefore diminished.

Observational studies allow studies to be performed that may be practically impossible to perform experimentally. For example, studies regarding body condition scores and fertility in cattle would be very expensive to study by experiment, yet relatively inexpensive to study by observational designs. This type of study is often used to investigate risk factors in disease, for example the development of urolithiasis and different types of cat food. There are three broad groups of observational studies: cohort, cross-sectional and case–control.

### 5.5.1   Cohort studies

A cohort study is a study in which animals exposed to a putative causal factor are followed over time, and compared with another group who are not exposed to that factor. The two groups are equally monitored for specific outcomes. Alternatively, two different treatments may be compared. Both groups contain animals which have the disease under investigation, and each group receives one of the two treatments (figure 5.6). This type of study allows comparison of risk and intervention. For example, dogs with an amputated hind leg could be monitored for the development of osteoarthritis in the remaining hind leg over a 24-month period. These animals would be compared with a group of healthy dogs. Matching the affected group to the control group is important to reduce any variables other than the factor of interest between the groups.

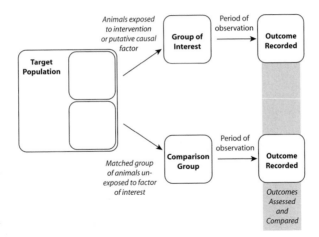

**Fig. 5.6**    A schematic representation of a cohort study

*Advantages*

- Cohort studies are generally preferred to case–control studies as they are statistically more reliable
- They are also cheaper than RCTs
- Compared with case–control studies they can establish the timing and sequence of events
- In prospective studies data collection can be standardised in comparison to the use of historical records.

*Disadvantages*

- Blinding and identifying a matched control group to minimise other variables can be difficult
- Cohort studies are not as reliable as the RCT as the two groups may differ in ways other than the variable under study
- Cohort studies can take a long time to complete, and there may be a loss of participants (drop out bias)
- They are not useful for rare diseases as it will be difficult to recruit sufficient patients.

### 5.5.2    Cross-sectional survey

The data can be used to determine a relationship between exposure to a factor and presence of disease. A representative sample of the whole population is sampled. Within the sample two groups are identified, usually dividing the group into those animals with a specified disease and those without. Identical sets of parameters are then recorded for the two groups (figure 5.7). The strength

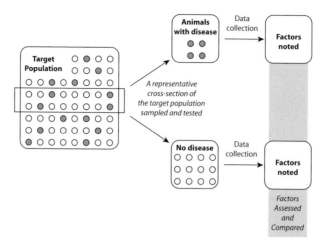

**Fig. 5.7**   A schematic representation of a cross-sectional study

of the relationship between the disease and the parameter can then be expressed as an odds ratio. This is the only type of study that can yield true prevalence rates.

*Advantages*

- They are relatively cheap to perform
- They present very few ethical problems.

*Disadvantages*

- No evidence of temporal relationships can be obtained from these studies, and so it is difficult to distinguish between cause and effect. Only association and lack of causation can be determined. Although combining our understanding of disease processes they can produce quite strong circumstantial evidence for causation
- They are studies that generate hypotheses rather than test hypotheses.

### 5.5.3   *Case–control studies*

Animals which have developed a disease condition are identified, and their exposure to suspected causal or risk factors is compared with that of a control group who do not have the disease (figure 5.8). Information regarding exposure is historical.

Risk factors may be investigated using this type of study by using a questionnaire.

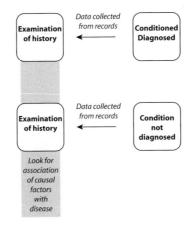

**Fig. 5.8** A schematic representation of a case–control study

For example, the diets of dogs with osteochondritis dessicans (OCD) could be compared with that of dogs that do not have OCD, and their dietary and exercise histories recorded for a possible link. However, just because there is a statistical relationship between a risk factor and a condition, it does not necessarily mean that there is a causal relationship. Case–control studies can also be used to provide evidence of whether an intervention has been effective or not. The results are expressed as odds ratios. Absolute risk cannot be determined.

## Advantages

- The main advantages are that they are quick to perform and do not require special methods to conduct
- They are generally inexpensive and may be the only way in which rare conditions or those with a long incubation period can be realistically studied
- They can be used to evaluate interventions as well as associations.

## Disadvantages

- Case–control studies are less reliable than either RCTs or cohort studies as it is difficult to match the control group and eliminate confounding variables
- It is not possible to calculate true incidence/prevalence and relative risk
- They are useful to formulate hypotheses that can be tested using study designs higher up on the hierarchy, such as cohort or RCTs.
- Data is collected retrospectively and elements of data may be missing or of poor quality.

## 5.6   Diagnostic tests and screening tests

The two parameters that describe a test are the sensitivity and the specificity. The sensitivity is the frequency of a positive result in the animals that have a specified disease. The specificity is the frequency of a negative test in animals that do not have the disease. From this information the likelihood ratio for the presence of the diseases for a given result can be generated (see Chapter 6).

To determine the sensitivity of a test, a group of animals with the disease for which the test is being evaluated is required. Not only should they have the disease, but they should represent the various stages of the disease that will be encountered in the population it is intended for. In order to confirm that these animals have the disease a gold (reference) standard test is required that is 'Always right', i.e. has a specificity and sensitivity of 100%. This is often difficult to achieve (or to be sure of). Post-mortem examinations are frequently used as a gold standard. The second group required is to determine the specificity. This group must not have the disease and, ideally, should represent the population on which the test is to be used, i.e. contain the same proportions of healthy animals and the same prevalence of other diseases. So although the sensitivity and specificity are independent of the prevalence of the diseases being tested the groups should represent the population for which it is going to be used. It is important that confidence intervals are determined for the results. The larger the number of animals in the groups, the narrower the confidence intervals will be.

## 5.7   Poorly controlled or uncontrolled trials

### 5.7.1   Comparisons between groups at different times

Historical data from subjects that did not receive the treatment is used for comparison with the current experimental group. Historical controls often have poor outcomes and are rarely matched appropriately to the current treatment group. As a consequence these comparisons often show the test treatment in a favourable light, and should be viewed with caution, as there are many other variables that may have affected the result.

### 5.7.2   Comparisons between different places

If league tables of performance and outcomes were introduced into the veterinary profession as a means of auditing competency there would be a grave danger that, in the absence of a detailed demographic analysis, the results would be misinterpreted. It is essential that scientific method is applied to this method of reporting, even if it means rejecting all the conclusions. These tables may be able to highlight areas of potential concern, but without more detailed scientific validation the evidence supplied by such information is usually weak.

### 5.7.3   n = 1 trials (the 'treat and see' method)

All veterinary surgeons have used the 'treat and see' approach as a valid methodology in the treatment of individual patients. A good example is the treatment of osteoarthritis in the aging dog, where there is a wide selection of treatment options. Although evidence is available in the literature, individual patient circumstances and variation in response sometimes means that the best treatment is not always obvious. In order to select the best treatment for an individual patient a trial of different therapies used sequentially is performed on the animal in question. In order to increase the objectivity of this exercise, good patient records, using well-defined descriptors, should be used to identify the best treatment, rather than relying on memory.

### 5.7.4   Uncontrolled trials (before and after trials)

Some trials evaluate outcomes before and after an intervention has been introduced, and assume that the difference between them is solely due the intervention. This is a dangerous assumption as there are many factors that are time dependent.

Another form of uncontrolled study presents the outcomes and harm from a cohort of treated patients. This study cannot distinguish between the outcome with the treatment and that without the treatment, as the observations may just reflect the natural history of the disease rather than any effect of the treatment.

### 5.7.5   Non-random allocation trials

Bias is a major problem with non-randomised trials. True randomisation involves the use of a formal randomising method and should not be confused with the arbitrary assignment of animals to treatments. Selecting alternate cases for treatments, or using a different treatment on certain days of the week are examples of arbitrary selection and may introduce confounding factors, however unlikely it may seem. True randomisation is extremely easy to achieve and is only avoided as a result of ignorance or laziness.

## 5.8   Descriptive studies

Surveys, case series and case reports are different types of descriptive study.

### 5.8.1   Surveys

Surveys are descriptive studies applied to populations of animals. Properly conducted surveys are a form of cross-sectional study. Their objective is to provide data about the frequency of occurrence of a characteristic of interest such as disease prevalence or the presence of a risk factor. It is important that the sample population is representative of the target population and in this regard random sampling procedures are important to avoid bias.

### 5.8.2   Case series and case reports

A large proportion of the veterinary literature consists of case reports or case series (figure 5.9).

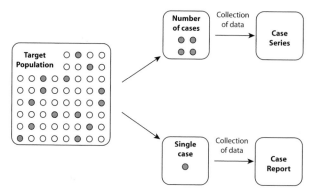

**Fig. 5.9**   A schematic representation of case series and case reports

A case report is a report on a single patient. A case series is a collection of case reports on the treatment of a condition, or a clinical description of a condition. A case report describes the presentation and/or course of a disease. It may be a novel presentation, or an undocumented course of a familiar disease, or a description of a rare disease. The purpose of the report is to present a particular history, clinical description, diagnosis, treatment or prognosis to the veterinary profession.

Case series can provide descriptive quantitative data. They are useful in identifying the range and the frequencies of presentations that may be encountered. Descriptions of treatments and associated potential risk factors should be viewed with extreme caution and used to generate hypotheses only.

Case series and case reports have no statistical validity since there is no control group but may be helpful if other sources of evidence are not available with regard to a rare condition. Case report and case series are not usually regarded as research, and are traditionally regarded as the lowest form of evidence. However, in the absence of other sources of information they have an important part to play in the acquisition of evidence.

*Advantages*

- Rare complications of interventions may be reported that may not be documented in other research trials
- New and emerging diseases may be first described as a case report, e.g. BSE
- They may serve as early indicators of novel developments, risks and diagnostic and therapeutic options
- Hypothesis generating not hypothesis proving.

*Disadvantages*

- The intervention described may not have influenced the outcome
- There may be harm attached to the intervention
- The description may be atypical of the rare disease
- There may be a publication bias, in that promising or interesting interventions are published, whereas less interesting or unpromising ones are not
- Conclusions from these reports should be interpreted with maximum caution.

## Further reading

Dahoo, I.R. and Waltner-Toews, D. (1985) Interpreting clinical research: Part I. General considerations. *Compendium of Continuing Education* **7**(9), S474–7.

Dahoo, I.R. and Waltner-Toews, D. (1985) Interpreting clinical research: Part II. Descriptive and experimental studies. *Compendium of Continuing Education* **7**(9), S513–19.

Dahoo, I.R. and Waltner-Toews, D. (1985) Interpreting clinical research: Part III. Observational studies and interpretation of results. *Compendium of Continuing Education* **7**(9), S605–13.

McGovern, D.P.B., Valori, R.M., Summerskill, W.S.M. and Levi, M. (2001) *Key Topics in Evidence-Based Medicine.* BIOS Scientific Publications Ltd, Oxford.

## Review questions

Answers on page 205

**1** *A descriptive study:*

(a) Contains a control group
(b) Explains the cause of a disease
(c) Records events only
(d) Randomly allocates animals to different treatments
(e) Is a qualitative not a quantitative study.

**2** *Which of the following statements about case reports is false?*

(a) A case report is usually about a rare condition
(b) A case report usually describes the clinical signs of a condition
(c) A case report provides strong evidence for the cause of a condition
(d) Case reports may give atypical descriptions
(e) Case reports are useful as an early warning system of new and emerging diseases.

**3** *Which of the following are explanatory experimental studies?*

(a) Randomised control trials
(b) Clinical trials, cross-over studies, case series
(c) Cohort, cross-sectional studies, case–control studies
(d) Case reports, surveys
(e) Cross-sectional studies and cohort studies.

**4** *Which of the following are observational studies?*

(a) Randomised control trials
(b) Clinical trials, cross-over studies, case series
(c) Cohort, cross-sectional studies, case–control studies
(d) Case reports, surveys
(e) Cross-sectional studies and cohort studies.

**5** *Which of the following are descriptive studies?*

(a) Randomised control trials
(b) Clinical trials, cross-over studies, case series
(c) Cohort, cross-sectional studies, case–control studies
(d) Case reports and case series
(e) Cross-sectional studies and cohort studies.

**6** *The difference between a meta-analysis and a systematic review is:*

(a) The number of studies included
(b) In a meta-analysis the data from the studies are combined for statistical analysis, in a systematic review they are not
(c) Systematic reviews provide stronger evidence than meta-analyses
(d) The type of statistics applied to the data from the studies
(e) There is no difference.

**7** *Select the sequence of study type that goes from strongest to weakest in providing valid evidence (the hierarchy of evidence).*

(a) Randomised controlled trial, case–control study, case report
(b) Randomised controlled trial, case report, case–control study
(c) Systematic review, case studies, cohort study
(d) Meta-analysis, case studies, systematic review
(e) Meta-analysis, cohort study, randomised controlled trial.

**8** *The power of an experiment indicates:*

(a) The cost of the experiment
(b) The ability of the study to demonstrate a difference
(c) The difficulty of performing the experiment
(d) The dose of the drug used
(e) The concentration of the drug being used.

**9** *Which of the following best describes the factors influencing the power of the study?*

(a) Size of the study groups or population
(b) The study design
(c) The natural variation in the parameters being measured
(d) The magnitude of the effect of the intervention
(e) All of the above.

**10** *A clinical trial differs from a laboratory study because:*

(a) Statistical analysis of the data is required
(b) A comparison of two groups is performed
(c) Animals in their natural environment are used
(d) The allocation of the animals to the two groups is under the control of the researcher
(e) Clinical outcomes should be measured.

# 6

# APPRAISING THE EVIDENCE

The aim of this chapter is to provide the reader with basic guidelines for determining the validity and the relevance of clinical studies. This evaluation is obtained by answering the questions, 'Is it true?' and 'Is it relevant to my question/patient?'

After reading this chapter the reader should be able to:

- Appraise articles on veterinary therapy
- Appraise articles about diagnosis
- Appraise articles on aetiology
- Appraise articles on prognosis.

84

## 6.1 Some introductory concepts

Although the authors do not wish to burden readers with a lot of statistical or epidemiological theory which may be better obtained from specialist textbooks (listed in the bibliography), there are a few important concepts which require an introduction.

### 6.1.1 The importance of statistics

While it is not necessary to become an expert in statistics in order to appraise the literature one does have to acknowledge its absolute and fundamental importance.

Why is it so important?

It is part of the human condition that we view things subjectively. We instinctively find some information hard to believe, while we are prepared to believe other 'facts' without proper scrutiny or evidence.

It might help to consider the following (often used) example.

A lecturer is addressing 31 students and offers to bet £10 that two of the students in the room share the same birthday.

Given that there are 365 days in the year and only 31 students this would seem like a rash bet. To anyone not familiar with this statistical phenomenon their instinct is that the chance of any two students having the same birthday is certainly less than 0.5 (1 in 2). The actual chance of this happening is 0.73 (approximately 3 in 4) which means that for every 4 times the lecturer makes this bet (with a new class of students of course) the lecturer will win 3 times. (Readers may wish to know how this was calculated, or may wish to attempt a solution themselves. Hint: it is easier to calculate the chance of two students not having the same birthday. The solution is given at the end of the chapter.)

It doesn't require a leap of the imagination to consider the researcher looking at the results of a clinical trial showing a large difference between the treated and non-treated animals and thinking that with such obvious results, a statistical analysis is unnecessary. Sadly, statistical analysis is always necessary.

The complexity of clinical trials and the small scale of veterinary research in comparison with the medical world often require skilled statistical consideration. This represents a problem to the researchers on the one hand but an even bigger problem to the practising veterinary surgeon on the other. It is unreasonable to expect every veterinary surgeon to be able to detect the inappropriate use of statistics and so we must rely on the quality of peer review. Many journals now use a specialised statistical reviewer or editor to check the statistics included in papers. For this, and other reasons, any paper appearing in a non-peer-reviewed journal will require special scrutiny before its results are considered as evidence.

There is a hackneyed saying in the statistical world that 'If you torture the numbers long enough they'll eventually cough up a result'. So just because a paper reports a statistically significant result it doesn't make it especially valid, it doesn't even guarantee that it is true. At the minimum level that most journals accept (<0.05) it means that if the experiment was repeated 20 times and there was no effect to be seen, then on one occasion you might expect to see the results reported in the paper just as a result of natural variation, or coincidence. In other words, the reported phenomenon may just be a 1 in 20 chance event.

### 6.1.2 Likelihood: probability and odds

Another concept, used extensively during the appraisal process, which merits a brief introduction, is likelihood. Readers will already understand that likelihood is an expression of the certainty or uncertainty that an outcome will occur. Two common descriptors of likelihood are used: probability and odds.

The most widely used descriptor is probability. A probability of 1 (or 100%) indicates absolute certainty that an event will occur, and a probability of 0 (or 0%) a certainty that it won't. Values between 0 and 1 represent various degrees of uncertainty.

Odds describe likelihood as a ratio of the chances of an event occurring to the chances of it not occurring. We may be most familiar with odds in gambling terms. The bookmakers will place a horse at 1 to 10 odds because they believe it less likely to win than a horse they place at 1 to 2. Odds can be expressed as single figures by dividing the first figure by the second figure in the ratio (thus 1 to 10 becomes 0.1). If an event is more likely to occur than not, the odds value will be greater than 1. When an event is just as likely to happen as not (i.e. the chance of a coin landing heads up) the probability is 0.5 (or 50%), and the odds are 1:1 (or 1, also known as 'evens').

We can convert probability into odds by using the following formula:

$$\text{Odds} = \frac{\text{probability}}{(1 - \text{probability})}$$

and we can convert odds (as a single figure) into probability with another formula:

$$\text{Probability} = \frac{1}{(1 + \text{odds})}$$

Where odds are given as a two-figure ratio a to b, or a:b (e.g. 2:3) the formula is:

$$\text{Probability} = \frac{a}{a + b}$$

The disadvantages with odds are that you can't use odds to express certainty (not normally a problem in the real world), and that they are not always well understood by those of us who aren't epidemiologists, actuaries or gamblers. The use of odds enables otherwise complex formulae (e.g. Bayes' theorem) to be reduced to simple calculations. Some clients also find that odds are a slightly more intuitive format than probabilities for comparing likelihoods, particularly when considering remote possibilities. For example, a risk of anaesthetic death with a probability of 0.9901 may be perceived as too remote to be considered, whereas a death of 1 to 100 is still unlikely, but a tangible risk nonetheless.

In conclusion we can say that life would be simpler if we standardised on probability as a measure of likelihood but for pragmatic reasons practitioners of EBVM need to become familiar with the use of both odds and probability. A more extensive description of this topic can be found in the first chapter of the EBM textbook written by Richard Gross (2001).

### 6.1.3   *Risk and uncertainty*

A final introductory topic is one that we, as a society, are increasingly bad at understanding. The majority of the problems we face revolve around the understanding and communication of uncertainty. Whether it is communicating with clients, ranking differentials, or understanding clinical trial results. As scientists we are never absolutely certain, but we should know what we are least uncertain about. Statistics can provide quantified risk values, and can even provide the risk of the risk value being wrong (i.e. the confidence limits). However, very few of us think or communicate in numbers. We are not computers. Consider, for a moment, what common English language terms could be used to describe the probability of the most likely diagnosis in list of differentials (figure 6.1).

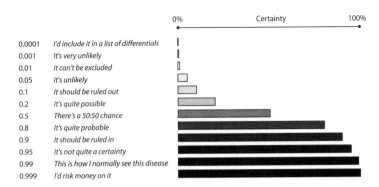

**Fig. 6.1**   A list of diagnostic probabilities illustrating the possible conversion of numerical values to linguistic terms

Through our own education we can understand the uncertainty and effectively appraise the evidence we use, and with this education and appropriate communication skills convey this information to clients and colleagues.

## 6.2  Appraising articles on veterinary therapy

In order to establish the validity of an article on therapy we need to ask the following questions:

- Was there a clearly defined research question?
- Was the assignment of patients to treatments randomised and was it blinded (i.e. owners and clinicians unaware of which treatment was used)?
- Were all the patients accounted for at the end of the study?
- Was there adequate follow-up?
- Were the groups for comparison treated equally throughout, and were they comparable?

In order to establish the importance of the result we need to have values for the following parameters:

$$\text{Relative risk reduction (RRR)} = \frac{\text{CER} - \text{EER}}{\text{CER}}$$

$$\text{Absolute risk reduction (ARR)} = \text{CER} - \text{EER}$$

$$\text{Number needed to treat (NNT)} = \frac{1}{\text{ARR}}$$

where CER is the control event rate and EER the experimental event rate (see below).

### 6.2.1  Is the study valid?

The bulk of this consideration requires us to satisfy some simple criteria, almost in the form of a checklist. If we answer these questions with a strong negative we should be prepared to disregard the results.

*Was there a clearly defined research question?*

What question was the study designed to answer? Was the question focused in terms of the population studied, the therapy tested, and the outcomes considered? For most clinical trials this will involve the comparison of one treatment against another, or ideally an untreated control group (sometimes we must be prepared to face the possibility that our patients get better in spite of our treatment rather than as a result of it!)

*Was the assignment of patients to treatments randomised and was it blinded (i.e. owners and clinicians unaware of which treatment was used)?*

In order to avoid any bias in the candidates selected for treatment and the way in which the treatments are assessed, randomisation and blinding are essential hence the importance of the randomised controlled trial (RCT). In a trial comparing surgical techniques double blinding may not be feasible but it is still important to try to ensure that the investigator assessing the outcome is unaware of the surgery used. True randomisation involves the use of a formal randomising strategy and should not be confused with the arbitrary assignment of patients to treatments. Selecting alternate patients for treatments, or using a different treatment on certain days of the week are examples of arbitrary selection and may introduce confounding factors, however unlikely it may seem. True randomisation is extremely easy to achieve and is only avoided as a result of ignorance or laziness.

Although placebo effect is an unlikely phenomenon in veterinary patients, it may become a factor when owners are providing some of the data on which the outcome is measured. Single-blinded trials are certainly acceptable in most circumstances.

*Were all the patients accounted for at the end of the study?*

When conducting a clinical trial in the 'real world' of veterinary practice it may be extremely difficult to ensure that every patient embarking on a treatment is kept in the trial to its conclusion. Road traffic accidents, clients moving, or owners withdrawing their animals from the study mean that some patients may not be accounted for at the end of the trial. A small well-documented attrition rate is acceptable, say 20% or less. However, unexplained losses or a high dropout rate should ring alarm bells. It is all too easy for frustrated investigators to remove patients from the trial data and influence the success, or failure rate of a particular treatment.

*Was there adequate follow-up?*

Studies must be long enough for any outcome to become evident. Clearly this will vary from treatment to treatment. Readers will use their clinical judgement to decide what is appropriate. Undesirable outcomes often take longer to manifest than desirable outcomes. Surgery trials should be subject to the same scrutiny as pharmacological trials.

*Were the groups for comparison treated equally throughout, and were they comparable?*

It is important that treatment groups are treated identically. It may be convenient to use the heifers in a milking herd as a negative control but they are not treated the same as the milking cows, nor are they a truly comparable group. Trials using veterinary hospital patients may use surgery patients as a negative control group; however, there may be a breed bias owing to the referral case load that a particular surgical team attracts. Breed, sex, and age distributions should always be indicated in a paper.

## 6.2.2   *Are the results important?*

From the report of the clinical trial we should learn the size of the treatment effect and the precision with which it has been detected.

The treatment effect observed in a study may be the result of:

- bias
- chance variation between the two groups
- the effect of the treatment.

We can rule out bias if we are satisfied that it was a valid study (as detailed above); we can reasonably disregard chance if the statistical analysis performed returns a *p* value of 0.05 or less (<0.01 is preferable, a 1:100 chance).

## 6.2.3   *Quantifying the risk of benefit or harm*

Both the clinician and the owner would probably like to know how likely a treatment is to produce an outcome. If one hundred identical dogs were treated, how many would get better? And how many would develop adverse reactions. These are called **event rates**.

The **control event rate** (CER) is the proportion of animals in the control group (either placebo, or a non-experimental treatment) demonstrating an effect.

The **experimental event rate** (EER) is the proportion of animals receiving the test treatment demonstrating an effect.

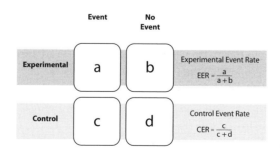

**Fig. 6.2**   A contingency table showing how EER and CER are calculated

*Relative risk reduction (RRR)*

Relative risk reduction is the proportion by which the treated group improves compared to the control group.

$$RRR = \frac{CER - EER}{CER}$$

*Absolute risk reduction (ARR)*

Absolute risk reduction is the absolute difference between the control and experimental group.

$$ARR = CER - EER$$

ARR is a more useful measure than RRR in most clinical situations. RRR removes consideration of the background risk so that when looking at a rare event a small difference in the treatment group produces the same RRR as a large difference when looking at a more common event.

Consider two different clinical situations. Two different diseases for which vaccination is effective. In the first disease 88% of unvaccinated animals develop the disease, and 15% of vaccinates. In the second disease 8.8% of unvaccinated animals develop the disease, which is reduced to 1.5% on vaccination.

|  | CER (unvaccinated) | EER (vaccinated) | ARR | RRR |
|---|---|---|---|---|
| Disease 1 | 0.88 (88%) | 0.15 (15%) | $0.88 - 0.15 = 0.73$ (73%) | $\dfrac{0.88 - 0.15}{0.88} = 83\%$ |
| Disease 2 | 0.088 (8.8%) | 0.015 (1.5%) | $0.088 - 0.015 = 0.073$ (7%) | $\dfrac{0.088 - 0.015}{0.088} = 83\%$ |

The two vaccines against the different diseases have identical relative risk reductions but the absolute benefits have a ten-fold difference.

*Number needed to treat (NNT)*

An extremely useful measure of benefit, which most of us find easy to understand, is the inverse of the absolute risk reduction. It tells us the number of patients we would have to treat in order to prevent one bad outcome.

$$NNT = \frac{1}{ARR}$$

In a paper by Olivry *et al.* (2002) the use of oral cyclosporine was compared with the use of prednisolone for the treatment of canine atopic dermatitis in an

RCT. In the results of the trial it was reported that there was a reduction in pruritis in 71% (10/14) of dogs treated with prednisolone and in 77% (10/13) dogs treated with cyclosporine. The ARR of pruritis resulting from the use of cyclosporine was 0.06 (77%–71%).

Therefore the NNT in order to achieve the relief of pruritis in one extra case is:

$$NNT = \frac{1}{0.06} = 16.7 \approx 17 \text{ dogs}$$

### 6.2.4   *Confidence intervals (CIs)*

We are used to seeing so-called 'error bars' on graphs included in scientific papers, and ranges given in tables. These are given because we need to have some indication of the certainty of the figure, or the likely range of figures we could expect from multiple repeats of the study. The most clinically useful example of these is the confidence interval. Any trial uses a sample taken from the entire possible population (i.e. some cats with renal failure rather than all cats with renal failure). The confidence interval takes into account the sampling error (as opposed to the statistical significance indicated by the *p* value), and it is often described as indicating clinical significance. For example, if 95% confidence intervals were given for red cell numbers in cats with renal failure, a veterinary surgeon in practice could expect 95 out of every 100 cats seen with renal failure to have red cell counts in that range. It is beyond the scope of this book to compare and contrast other methods of demonstrating expected ranges, but they are reported rarely in the veterinary literature at a time when their use in the medical literature is increasing rapidly. The usefulness of confidence intervals is their ability to set single values in perspective. An NNT of 7 with a 95% CI of 3 to 9 is clearly more useful than a NNT of 7 with a 95% CI of 3 to 28.

$$95\% \text{ CI on the ARR} = \pm 1.96 \times \sqrt{\frac{CER \times (1 - CER)}{\text{no. of control animals}} + \frac{EER \times (1 - EER)}{\text{no. of exper. animals}}}$$

If we apply this to the clinical trial results used as an example in Section 2.3 above we would calculate the following 95% CI for the ARR:

$$95\% \text{ CI on the ARR} = \pm 1.96 \times \sqrt{\frac{0.71 \times (1 - 0.71)}{14} + \frac{0.77 \times (1 - 0.77)}{13}}$$

$$95\% \text{ CI on the ARR} = \pm 1.96 \times 0.168 = \pm 0.33 \text{ or } 33\%$$

Clearly the confidence intervals on the risk reduction are greater than the risk reduction itself and so we are forced to conclude that the evidence for using cyclophosphamide over prednisolone is unproven in the results from this trial (the small group size was the problem in this case).

The 95% CI on an NNT = 1/(the 95% CI on its ARR)

When a confidence crosses the line of no difference (i.e. the point at which it becomes disadvantageous), then we can conclude that the results are not clinically useful.

### Relative risk (RR)

Relative risk is the ratio of the experimental event rate to the control event rate and is used to quantify the difference in risk between the two groups.

$$RR = \frac{EER}{CER}$$

An RR below 1 shows there is less chance of the event happening in the experimental group, and an RR above 1 shows there is a greater chance. Again there is no reference to the baseline risk, and therefore the absolute benefit to be gained.

## 6.2.5 Making a decision about therapy

An evidence-based approach to deciding if a treatment is effective for a patient involves the following steps:

(1)  Frame the clinical question.
(2)  Search for the evidence concerning the efficacy of one or more treatments.
(3)  Assess the methodology used to perform the trial.
(4)  Determine the NNT of the therapy(ies).
(5)  Assess the applicability to the patient (adjust NNT if necessary).
(6)  Incorporate the patient's values and client preferences into deciding a course of action.

## 6.3 Appraising articles on veterinary diagnosis

In order to establish the validity of an article on diagnosis we need to ask the following questions:

- Was there a clearly defined question?
- Was the presence or absence of the target disorder confirmed with a reliable and accurate test ('a gold standard' test)?
- Was the test evaluated on a relevant or appropriate population?
- Was the condition confirmed in all cases?
- Can the test be used in your practice, on this patient?

In order to establish the importance of the result we need to have values for the following parameters:

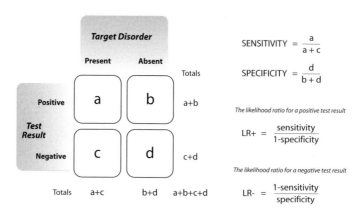

**Fig. 6.3**　A contingency table showing how results of a diagnostic test can be analysed

$$\text{Sensitivity} = \frac{a}{a+c}$$

$$\text{Specificity} = \frac{d}{b+d}$$

Likelihood ratio for a positive test result,

$$\text{LR}+ = \frac{\text{sensitivity}}{1-\text{specificity}}$$

Likelihood ratio for a negative test result,

$$\text{LR}- = \frac{1-\text{sensitivity}}{\text{specificity}}$$

### 6.3.1　Is the study valid?

*Was there a clearly defined question?*

- Exactly which question was the study designed to answer? Was there adequate focus on the condition or test evaluated? Is the population selected appropriate to your patient's species (or possibly breed)?
- Was the presence or absence of the target disorder confirmed with a reliable and accurate test ('a gold standard' test)?
- How did the investigators establish whether or not the animals had the disease? They may have used a number of criteria including existing diagnostic tests or procedures. Were these validated? If clinical expertise was used, were the individuals concerned blinded as to the test results? Beware of cross-species assumptions.

*Was the test evaluated on a relevant or appropriate population?*

Was the test used on an outbred population of animals? Were the animals tested appropriate to a practice population in terms of breed, husbandry, age, and so on? Could there have been other diseases affecting the results?

*Was the condition confirmed in all cases?*

All patients should have the condition or disease confirmed by use of the 'gold standard' test. If there are exceptions they should be considered carefully for sources of potential bias. It may be that a post-mortem diagnosis is used with only a proportion of animals; if so, how confident can we be in the diagnosis of the remaining animals?

*Can the test be used in your practice, on this patient?*

There may be obvious reasons in terms of cost, equipment, skills, or invasiveness, why this test is inappropriate for a particular client, patient or veterinary practice.

### 6.3.2   Are the results important?

The two questions that we want to know when we have used a diagnostic test are:

- What does a positive result mean for our patient?
- What does a negative result mean for our patient?

There are many different (and possibly confusing) ways in which the accuracy of a test may be reported because each test is attempting to identify two populations: the animals free of the disease, and those animals with the disease. Measures of accuracy look at four different possibilities:

(1)   The test can be positive in animals with the disease (a true positive result).
(2)   The test can be positive in animals free of the disease (a false positive).
(3)   The test can be negative in animals with the disease (a false negative).
(4)   The test can be negative in animals free of the disease (a true negative).

Ideally we want to maximise the instances of (1) and (4), while minimising the instances of (2) and (3).

**Sensitivity** is the proportion of diseased animals with a positive result.

**Specificity** is the proportion of animals without the disease with a negative result.

We combine these measures into the indicators of the overall efficiency of a test by calculating **likelihood ratios** (LRs). Likelihood ratios enable us to convert a pre-test probability of disease to a post-test probability (thus answering our two important questions above).

The positive likelihood ratio is the ratio of the proportion of positive-test animals who have the disease (sensitivity) to the proportion of positive-test animals who do not have the disease (1 − specificity). The negative likelihood ratio similarly gives us the ratio of false negatives (1 − sensitivity) to true negatives (specificity).

It is important to realise that the sensitivity and specificity (and thus LRs) are absolute measures of a test's performance; however, the post-test probability is determined by the amount of disease present in the population in the first place, the pre-test probability. The pre-test probability is numerically the same as the prevalence of the disease (conceptually, pre-test probability applies to an individual, whereas prevalence applies to a population). Good disease prevalence data is rare in veterinary practice and a paper may describe the results of a test in experimental animals. A veterinary practitioner may be able to produce post-test probabilities by factoring prevalence data from practice records or even by estimating based on recent experience. Sometimes the prevalence data used by the paper describing the test may be appropriate for your patient.

From all this, it is clear that we need to know how well the test performs (i.e. sensitivity and specificity) and prevalence data in order to answer the two important questions. What does a positive result mean for our patient? What does a negative result mean for our patient?

Consider an example of a commercially available FeLV ELISA test whose diagnostic performance was described in a paper by Hartmann *et al.* (2001). The samples tested were from 800 apparently healthy cats prior to FeLV vaccination. The reference standard used was the isolation of the FeLV from blood.

### For a positive result

Post-test odds = pre-test odds × likelihood ratio = 0.099 × 45.5 = 4.5 (see figure 6.4)

(we'll get 1 false positive for every 4.5 true positives, from a total of 5.5 cats testing positive, or because we deal in whole animals 2 false positives for every 9 true positives).

$$\text{Post-test probability} = \frac{\text{post-test odds}}{1 + \text{post-test odds}} = \frac{4.5}{5.5} = 82\%$$

(this cat has an 82% chance of having FeLV, 18 in every 100 will be false positives).

### For a negative result

Pre-test odds (for presence of the disease) = 0.099

Post-test odds = pre-test odds × likelihood ratio = 0.099 × 0.09 = 0.0089

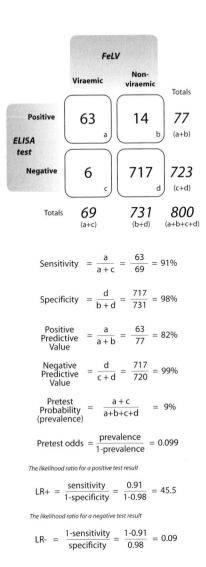

**Fig. 6.4** A contingency table analysing the results of an ELISA test for FelV

(we'll get 0.0089 false negatives, from a total of 1.0089 animals testing negative, or in whole animal terms, 89 for every 10 000, which is approximately 1 for every 112 true negatives).

$$\text{Post-test probability of disease} = \frac{0.0089}{1 + 0.0089} = 0.0088 \approx 1\%$$

(this cat has a 1% chance of having FeLV, approximately 1 out of 100 will be false negatives).

These figures enable us to provide clients with reliable information rather than mere opinion when we give them the results. If we assume our client's animal is represented by the population referred to in the paper, and that the prevalence of disease is similar, then we can be 82% sure that the cat has FeLV. When we get a negative result we can be 99% sure that the cat is FeLV free at the time the sample was taken.

If the prevalence of FeLV in your practice was 18%, the figures would change to reveal that 91% of the positive testing cats, and approximately 2% of cats testing negative, would actually be viraemic. Readers could take the opportunity to attempt the calculations themselves, or for approximate determination use the nomogram in figure 6.5.

### 6.3.3   SpPin and SnNout

Although sensitivity and specificity alone do not reveal the whole diagnostic picture, the mnemonics SpPin and SnNout are worth remembering. Using a specific test (Sp), getting a positive result (P) means we should rule that diagnosis in (in) – **SpPin**. Using a sensitive test (Sn), getting a negative result (N) means we can rule that diagnosis out (out) – **SnNout**.

### 6.3.4   Making a decision about a diagnostic test

An evidence-based approach to interpreting a diagnostic test for a patient involves the following steps:

(1)   Formulate the clinical question.
(2)   Search for the evidence concerning the accuracy of the test.
(3)   Appraise the methodology used.
(4)   Determine the likelihood ratios for the test.
(5)   Estimate the pre-test probability of disease for the patient.
(6)   Calculate the post-test probability using the likelihood ratio and the pre-test probability (use of the nomogram in figure 6.5 avoids the use of arithmetic).
(7)   Form a decision on which test to use based on whether or not it will influence therapy decisions and the clients' concerns.

## 6.4   Appraising articles on harm or aetiology

In order to establish the validity of an article on aetiology or harm we need to ask the following questions:

- Was there a well-defined research question?
- Were the groups of animals clearly defined and comparable?

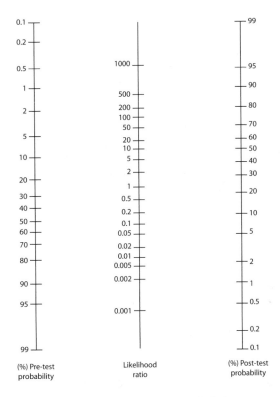

**Fig. 6.5** Nomogram for determining post-test probabilities. To use the nomogram position a ruler (or other straight edge) to connect the estimate of an animal's pre-test probability of disease (on the left-hand scale), to the point on the central scale that corresponds to the likelihood ratio of the test. The post-test probability can now be read off the right-hand scale

- Was the exposure to factors and the clinical outcomes measured identical in both groups?
- Were the animals followed up for long enough, and thoroughly enough?
- Does the suggested cause make sense?

In order to establish the importance of the result we need to have values for the following parameters:

In an RCT or cohort study:

Relative risk, RR

In a case–control study:

Odds ratio, OR

### 6.4.1   *Is the study valid?*

When looking at harm (adverse effects of therapy) or disease aetiology, investigators usually use prospective cohort studies or retrospective case–control studies (see Chapter 5).

*Was there a well-defined research question?*

Good science is generated from asking the right questions. Is it clear what question the research was designed to answer and was it focused? Is the population relevant to your veterinary practice?

*Were the groups of animals clearly defined and comparable?*

When looking at harm the study must establish that the two groups are similar in every way other than exposure to the putative cause of the harm. Experimental studies might achieve this through randomisation. Is there sufficient evidence that there is no selection bias in either group that may introduce confounders? Typically the owners of animals referred to veterinary schools or veterinary hospitals are a self-selecting group of concerned and assiduous individuals. Comparing their animals with animals from a rescue shelter, for example, would clearly be inappropriate.

*Was the exposure to factors and the clinical outcomes measured identical in both groups?*

The degree of investigation and the methods used should be identical for both groups.

*Were the animals followed up for long enough, and thoroughly enough?*

Follow-up should be adequate to allow long-term as well as short-term problems to manifest themselves. A dropout rate of greater than 20% should be regarded as a serious flaw as these animals may have very different outcomes from those remaining in the study.

*Does the suggested cause make sense?*

It is likely that 'non-sensical' results will be spotted by the scrutineers of the paper (indeed it may be difficult to get certain 'interesting' results published); however, look out for the following:

- Is it evident that exposure preceded the outcome? It should be clear that the exposure is not just a marker of pre-existing disease.

- Is there a dose–response gradient? Greater exposure to a factor (either in amount, or over time) might be expected to create a greater degree of harm.
- Dechallenge–rechallenge studies can be used to demonstrate that harm reduces when exposure is halted, and returns with subsequent re-exposure. Cross-over studies can be used to swap over the two groups in this way.
- Is the association consistent from study to study? There is a tendency in the veterinary literature for a single reporting of an adverse effect to rapidly become dogma. Properly executed systematic reviews help to put such findings in context. Sadly, too many book chapters and continuing education articles fail to do this.
- Does the association make biological sense? This should be used as a 'ruling in' question rather than necessarily a reason to rule it out. EBVM does not preclude an open mind although it does require a healthy scepticism.

### 6.4.2   Are the results important?

Having accepted the validity of a study we now look at the risk or odds of the adverse effect occurring with a particular treatment or exposure. If the risk is high because of a high association it will have greater clinical importance.

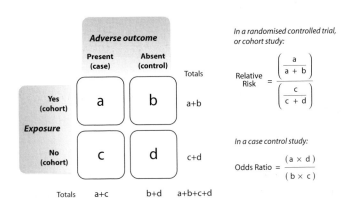

**Fig. 6.6**   A contingency table showing calculations of relative risk and odds ratio

In an RCT or cohort study:

$$\text{Relative risk, RR} = \frac{\left(\dfrac{a}{a+b}\right)}{\left(\dfrac{c}{c+d}\right)}$$

In a case–control study:

$$\text{Odds ratio, } OR = \frac{(a \times d)}{(b \times c)}$$

To calculate the **number needed to harm** (NNH) we require the OR and the **patients experimental event rate** (PEER)

$$NNH = \frac{[PEER \times (OR - 1)] + 1}{[PEER \times (OR - 1)] \times (1 - PEER)}$$

The relative merits of cohort and case–control studies are described in Chapter 5.

### 6.4.3 *Statistical analysis*

The range indicator of choice is the 95% confidence interval. If the range crosses the value of no difference (i.e. 1) it means that there may be no effect, or even a beneficial effect!

## 6.5 Appraising studies on prognosis

In order to establish the validity of an article on prognosis we need to ask the following questions:

- Is the sample representative?
    Were cases recruited at a common point in their illness?
    Did the study account for other important factors?
    Is the setting representative?
- Was the follow-up long enough to assess the clinical outcome?
- Was the follow-up complete?
- Were the outcomes measured blind?

In order to establish the importance of the result we need to have values for the following parameters:

- What is the risk of outcome over time?
- How precise are the estimates?

95% confidence intervals are $\pm 1.96$ times the standard error (SE) of the measure. SE of a proportion:

$$SE = \sqrt{\frac{p \times (1 - p)}{n}}$$

Although veterinary studies purely on prognosis are relatively uncommon there is a considerable amount of data on the prognosis of certain conditions in the literature. Most veterinary prognostic data comes from papers on therapy, which has been covered above. However, when the prognostic aspects of such studies are read, additional appraisal is required. When clients are faced with emotional and potentially expensive decisions we can help make their decisions better informed by providing what information we can. When seeking information about a patient's likely prognosis over time, the most useful data comes from a longitudinal cohort study.

### 6.5.1   Is the study valid?

*Is the sample representative?*

Does the study clearly define a group of patients within which your patient could be represented? Did the study use clear inclusion and exclusion criteria?

*Were cases recruited at a common point in their illness?*

The methods section of the paper should include a clear description of the stage and timing of the illness being considered. To obtain a complete understanding of the prognostic factors, an ideal study would include patients from the onset of disease up until the animal's death. This is impossible to achieve in non-experimental studies but serious bias can result from over-representation of early stage, or late stage disease in the cohort.

*Did the study account for other important factors?*

The investigators should examine any other possible factor that might influence outcomes. Factors such as breed, husbandry, sex, age, and concurrent disease may influence the measured outcome of disease. The population under study may not be exposed to factors experienced by your patient. Clinical judgement (as ever) enables us to factor in (or out) aspects relevant to a particular case.

*Is the setting representative?*

Client compliance with treatment may be greater with patients from a referral practice than in clients from general practice. Levels of aftercare or husbandry will vary markedly between different clinical situations with the wide variety of species and breeds seen in veterinary practice.

*Was the follow-up long enough to assess the clinical outcome?*

It is important that sufficient time for adequate follow-up is provided. There is little point in informing clients of the good immediate prognosis for their animal if long-term harmful effects subsequently appear. In general, chronic diseases require longer follow-up.

*Was the follow-up complete?*

When patients disappear from the cohort we want to know why. Greater than a 20% loss should be seen as a considerable potential for the introduction of bias. Were the outcomes measured blind?

### 6.5.2    *Are the results important?*

What is the risk of outcome with time? Outcomes may be presented in three ways:

- Proportion (percentage) of animals which survive at a particular time
- The length of time it takes for half the animals to have the outcome (the median survival)
- A survival curve, which depicts the proportion of animals from the original study sample which have not yet had the specified outcome.

Survival curves provide the additional information of temporal changes of risk over time.

*How precise is the prognostic information?*

In order to account for sampling error, 95% confidence intervals should be provided. These represent the range in which we can be 95% certain that the true value lies. This range should be considered when providing a prognosis for an individual patient. A wide range indicates that the study had insufficient numbers to provide useful information.

For normally distributed data CI = 1.96 × SE either side of the value.

$$SE = \sqrt{\frac{p \times (1 - p)}{n}}$$

## References and further reading

Badenoch, D. and Heneghan, C. (2002) *Evidence-based Medicine Toolkit.* BMJ Books, London. [A considerable proportion of this chapter was based on the structure of this small book which can be highly recommended to reader.]

Gross, R. (2001) *Decisions and Evidence in Medical Practice.* Mosby, St Louis.

Hartmann, K., Werner, R.M., Egberink, H. and Jarrett, O. (2001) Comparison of six in-house tests for the rapid diagnosis of feline immunodeficiency and feline leukaemia virus infections. *Vet Rec* **149**(11), 317–20.

Olivry, T., Rivierre, C., Jackson, H.A., Murphy, K.M., Davidson, G. and Sousa, C.A. (2002) Cyclosporine decreases skin lesions and pruritus in dogs with atopic dermatitis: a blinded randomized prednisolone-controlled trial. *Vet Dermatol* **13**(2), 77–87.

## Review questions

Answers on page 205

**1** *What is the odds equivalent of a 20% probability?*

   (a)  0.2
   (b)  1:5
   (c)  0.25
   (d)  1:4

**2** *Which of the following is the correct formula for the number needed to treat?*

   (a)  $NNT = \dfrac{1}{ARR}$

   (b)  $NNT = \dfrac{1}{RRR}$

   (c)  $NNN = \dfrac{1}{CER}$

   (d)  $NNN = \dfrac{1}{PEER}$

**3** *Which of the following best define the terms sensitivity and specificity?*

   (a)  Sensitivity is the proportion of diseased animals with a positive result.
      Specificity is the proportion of animals without the disease with a negative result.
   (b)  Sensitivity is the proportion of animals without the disease with a negative result.
      Specificity is the proportion of diseased animals with a positive result.
   (c)  Sensitivity is the proportion of true positives testing negative for the disease
      Specificity is the proportion of true negatives testing positive for the disease
   (d)  Sensitivity is the ratio of the true positives to the true negatives
      Specificity is the inverse of the sensitivity

**4** *What does the likelihood ratio for a negative test result tell us?*

   (a)  The likelihood of the animal being disease free, given a negative test result.
   (b)  The likelihood of the animal being disease free, given a positive test result.
   (c)  The likelihood of the animal having a disease, given a negative test result.
   (d)  The likelihood of the animal having a disease, given a positive test result.

**5** *How would you best use a diagnostic test with a high specificity, but a low sensitivity?*

   (a)  To rule a diagnosis out
   (b)  To rule a diagnosis in.

## Solution to the probability example used in Section 1

When calculating the likelihood of any two people in a group having the same birthday it is easier to calculate the probability that someone does not have a birthday on the same day as another.

Starting with the second person they have a 364/365 (we'll ignore leap years) chance of not sharing a birthday with the first person.

The third person now has two possible birthdays to match up with, so they have a 363/365 chance of not sharing a birthday with the other two.

The fourth person has three possible birthdays to match up with, so their chance of not sharing the day is 362/365.

This continues to the 31st person who has a 335/365 chance of sharing a birthday with the others.

So to calculate the chance that all the people in the group have unique birthdays we have to multiply the different possibilities together (just as we multiply a half by a half to derive the possibility of tossing a coin twice and getting the same result).

$$p \text{ of unique birthdays} = \frac{364}{365} \times \frac{363}{365} \times \frac{362}{365} \times \ldots \times \frac{365 - 30}{365} = 0.27$$

Therefore the probability of not finding a set of unique birthdays is $1 - 0.27 = 0.73$ or 73%.

An elegant description of the solution together with a graphic demonstration of the phenomenon can be found at the following website address: www-stat.stanford.edu/~susan/courses/s116/node50.html

# 7

# DIAGNOSIS

After reading this chapter the reader should be able to

- Describe which method of clinical examination they are using
- Describe hypothetico-deductive reasoning
- Describe the three principal methods of pattern recognition
- Understand deductive and inductive reasoning
- Understand abstraction and logic
- Draw, explain and justify the process of diagnosis and the decisions made from clinical examination to closure
- Identify information needs in the diagnostic process
- Understand how sets, Venn diagrams and Boolean algebra can be used to describe diseases.

## 7.1    Introduction

Veterinary surgeons collect, collate, search out, investigate, accumulate, record, discard and finally process a large amount of data into understandable information in order to form diagnostic hypotheses. The accuracy of the data is critical. Most errors result from a lack of thoroughness in data collection, and not from a lack of knowledge. Veterinary surgeons make many diagnostic decisions during the course of their daily practice. However, few of us are aware of the underlying mechanisms involved in making such diagnoses, other than to vaguely attribute such an ability to experience, art, or an encyclopaedic knowledge. The more experienced a person becomes, the more difficult it is to explain the process to a third party. However, without an understanding of the underlying mechanisms, the process remains intuitive. When the process is intuitive, it cannot be taught, and the process of clinical reasoning cannot be made explicit or audited.

An understanding of the diagnostic process enables information needs to be established, and the process monitored. By appreciating these strategies the clinician should be able to explain the steps that were taken during the clinical reasoning process. As we understand the structural framework to achieve a diagnosis, the process becomes less intuitive, and the process more efficient. Analysis of the clinical reasoning used in a case will enable the clinician, and others, to identify errors and improvements. Additional information needs required for the process can be defined and located. This chapter describes some of the methods used in the process of data acquisition, clinical reasoning, and dealing with uncertainties. Strategies that can be used to assist the clinician in the process of clinical reasoning are described.

There are two components to the process.

- The identification of clinical abnormalities and disease associated risk factors
- Clinical reasoning that generates a diagnosis or differential diagnoses.

They may occur, one after the other, when we arrive at a diagnosis following a complete clinical examination and taking a history, or they may be used alternately in a repeated cycle, during the process of hypothetico-deductive reasoning.

## 7.2    Definitions

It is worth considering the definitions of a number of familiar terms in the context of the analysis of diagnostic methodology. Although these definitions may seem somewhat tortuous, a degree of precision is necessary to avoid ambiguity or confusion.

A **disease** may be defined as 'The sum of the abnormal phenomena displayed by a group of living organisms in association with a common characteristic or set of characteristics by which they differ from the norm of their species in such a way as to place them at a biological or economic disadvantage' (Campbell *et al.*, 1979). ('Economic' was added by White (1988) for veterinary medicine.)

**Diagnosis** is a task of classification. The usual goal of the veterinary surgeon is to place the cluster of problems of a patient, or group of patients, into the appropriate disease category. This involves sorting out the most likely hypothesis or hypotheses from what is often a wide range of possibilities. It is the determination of disease, or diseases, producing the clinical abnormalities in the patient. It is an expression of the opinion about the nature of the disease in the animal. It is a mapping from a patient's data (normal and abnormal history, physical examination and laboratory data) to a knowledge of the disease state. This is sometimes known as knowledge coupling.

## 7.2.1 Types of diagnosis

There are several different types of classification of diagnosis dependent upon the stage in the diagnostic work up and the degree of certainty attached to a diagnosis. The following list is from Radostits *et al.* (2000).

*Differential*

- Group of plausible possibilities
- Usually 3–5
- Ranked or prioritised relative to their likelihood of occurrence
- Probability and rank may change with new information.

*Tentative*

Suspected diagnosis not confirmed, e.g. milk fever based upon history and clinical signs.

*Presumptive*

- Usually made with more confidence than a tentative diagnosis, but still not definitively confirmed
- Exclusion of other common causes of the clinical presentation.

*Definitive and aetiological*

The diagnosis is confirmed using specific tests (e.g. Negri bodies for rabies) or clinical presentations (e.g. spastic paresis).

*Pathoanatomic (pathophysiological)*

Based on pathological findings, e.g. a fractured femur, congestive heart failure.

*Open*

> There are too many differential diagnoses, which cannot be ranked, or the presentation does not fit any common condition. Often occurs in the early stages of disease or with rare diseases, which have a non-specific presentation.

*Undetermined*

> In many cases in first opinion practice, the clinical presentation may be mild and vague so that a diagnosis cannot be achieved without extensive epidemiological, clinical and laboratory investigations. The immediate needs for treatment may be addressed before proceeding with expensive, time consuming tests, particularly if the presentation is mild and of short duration. However, if the response to treatment is poor then more extensive investigations are justified.

## 7.3   The clinical examination: evidence for the presence of disease

The purpose of the clinical examination is to identify the clinical abnormalities that are present, and the risk factors that lead to manifestation of disease in the individual, or a population. Agreement between veterinary surgeons in the recognition of abnormalities is not total. Sometimes it may be difficult to be certain that a particular clinical phenomenon is present.

The clinical examination ideally proceeds through a number of steps:

- owner's complaint
- signalment of the patient
- history of the patient(s)
- history of the farm
- observation of the environment
- observation of the animal at a distance
- detailed observations of the animal
- examination of the animal
- further investigations.

From this information the following may be derived:

- the most likely cause
- the organs or systems involved
- the location of the lesion
- the type of lesion present
- the pathophysiological processes occurring
- the severity of the disease
- the epidemiology of the outbreak.

Without a proficient clinical examination and an accurate diagnosis, the following are likely to be suboptimal:

- the treatment
- control
- the prognosis
- the welfare of the patient(s).

There are several different approaches to the clinical examination:

- the complete examination
- the problem-orientated examination
- the general examination.

The *complete clinical examination* consists of checking for the presence or absence of all clinical abnormalities and predisposing disease risk factors. From this information a ranked list of differential diagnoses is deduced. This is a failsafe method, and ensures no abnormality or risk factor is missed. The exhaustive approach includes all routine laboratory tests as well. 'Collect everything about everything' is one way of describing this method. Consequently, this method can be expensive in terms of time and cost. It is the safest approach if concurrent problems in a patient are suspected. However, the amount of information can be overwhelming.

The *problem-orientated method* (hypothetico-deductive method) combines clinical examination and a preconceived list of differential diagnoses. The sequence of the clinical investigation is dictated by the differential diagnoses generated from the previous findings. This results in a limited, but focused examination. The success of the method relies heavily on the background knowledge of the clinician, and usually assumes that a single condition is responsible for the abnormalities. It is an approach that is highly motivating as there is a higher probability of identifying an abnormality.

Many clinicians begin their examination by performing a *general examination* consisting of a broad search for abnormalities. The system or region involved is identified, and then examined in greater detail using either a complete or a problem-orientated examination.

## 7.4   Hypothetico-deductive reasoning

Hypothetico-deductive reasoning is a highly flexible approach to problem solving. Medical and veterinary students begin to generate hypotheses, or differential diagnoses, early in their clinical examinations without specific training or prompting. The method uses alternately, a data-driven forward chaining (deduction or *a posteriori* approach), and then a backward chaining (induction or *a priori*) method. The initial hypotheses are derived from the primary data acquisition. Subsequent data collection is guided by the leading hypothesis and the competing hypotheses being considered. The leading hypothesis may change depending on the new data acquired and may prompt further investigation. The competing hypotheses are compared one by one with the leading hypothesis.

This process continues recursively until a critical level of confidence has been reached. The final step is usually the validation of the diagnosis (the process is shown as a flow diagram in figure 7.1). Hypothesis generation or recall is critical. A correct diagnosis cannot be made if it has not even been considered.

Aggregation or collation of the individual findings from the initial data may simplify the diagnostic process. For example, signs consistent with congestive heart failure may result in the veterinary surgeon seeking causes of congestive heart failure rather than causes for the component signs. The generation of the initial list of possible diagnoses is sometimes selected by using an individual piece of data as a pivotal or key sign. The list of differentials will then include all the diseases that contain that pivotal sign. The pivotal sign (or pivot) is usually a sign which can be confidently recognised as an abnormality resulting from disease (Blood and Brightling, 1988).

The refinement process includes discriminating between close competitors, pursuing highly likely but unproven possibilities, ruling out less likely competitors and occasionally invoking new hypotheses when additional, unexpected findings are obtained. Signs or tests with a high specificity and sensitivity are selected to confirm or rule out a diagnosis. Each piece of information is considered with respect to all hypotheses under consideration before a diagnostic judgement is made. Findings are not sought if they are not related to one of the diagnostic possibilities under consideration.

This method produces a very specific and highly efficient search for information. It generates a high level of motivation in the clinician when compared with the use of a complete clinical examination as a first approach. The sign being investigated has a higher probability of being found when compared with a complete clinical examination. Complete clinical examinations yield a higher proportion of negative findings, which may induce a reduction in abnormality recognition due to investigator fatigue.

The number of hypotheses under consideration at any one time is usually four or five with a maximum of six or seven.

The recall of possible diagnoses and the ranking of competing hypotheses use a crucial function called pattern recognition which is described in Section 7.6.

## 7.5   The diagnostic process

Data processing is the method by which the database of information is transformed into diagnostic hypotheses or differential diagnoses. The precision of the data processing is critical. The complete or exhaustive method of data collection uses the sequence 1, 2, 3 and 5 illustrated below. The hypothetico-deductive method uses steps 1 to 5.

The steps of the diagnostic process are:

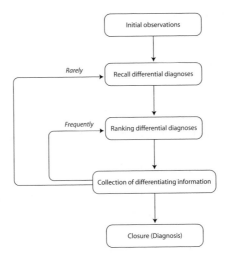

**Fig. 7.1** A schematic representation of the hypothetico-deductive diagnostic process

**Step 1**: Collection of data (clinical examination, laboratory tests).
**Step 2**: The recall of possible differential diagnoses (hypotheses).

Hypothesis generation (recall) is an important function, as the correct diagnosis cannot be made if it is not considered. The absence of a finding common to many diseases leads to a greater reduction of the differential diagnoses than the absence of a finding specific to a single disease. Confining the search to conditions consistent with the age, sex, breed, and class of animal (signalment) will also reduce the number of conditions to consider.

The recall strategies may include the recall of:

- diseases which contain all the signs observed
- diseases which contain only the signs you are confident about
- diseases for each sign observed
- diseases which contain most of the signs observed
- diseases which contain an important sign
- common diseases only.

**Step 3**: Ranking of competing differential diagnoses.

Pattern recognition is the process enabling a list of ranked differential diagnoses to be generated from the list of abnormalities. Three principal methods may be used:

- pattern matching
- probabilities
- pathophysiological reasoning.

**Step 4**: Further investigations to enable differentiation of the competing hypotheses.

Go back to step 1 if there are strongly competing differential diagnoses. Go to step 5 if the diagnosis is confirmed, as a result of evidence strongly in favour of a particular diagnosis.

**Step 5**: Closure (diagnosis).

Some of these steps are discussed in more detail below.

## 7.6   Recall and ranking

The process of recall and ranking requires a method of **pattern recognition**. Pattern recognition is the process leading to the generation of a list of ranked differential diagnoses from a list of abnormalities.

There are three broad categories of pattern recognition: pattern matching, probabilities, and pathophysiological reasoning.

### 7.6.1   *Pattern matching*

Pattern matching is a familiar cerebral process. When we notice someone, we instantly recognise a familiar face, a partially familiar face, or fail to recognise a stranger. The clinical signs observed are compared to profiles or descriptions of diseases we hold in our memory. The differential diagnosis list is constructed according to which of the disease profiles most closely match the clinical signs.

The pattern matching process may be restricted to common diseases in the initial hypothesis generation. If the closeness of the match deteriorates after obtaining additional data, the pattern matching may be extended to less common diseases. Pattern matching ability will increase with experience, as the archive in memory will be more complete and accurate.

### 7.6.2   *Probabilities*

A probability is computed using Bayes' theorem which requires:

- The prevalence of the diseases in the population
- The frequency of occurrence of the clinical signs observed within those diseases.

The differential list is then constructed from the disease probabilities.

*Conditional dependence and conditional independence of observations*

In most cases conditional independence of the signs is assumed and this can be an inaccurate assumption. Conditional independence simply means that it is assumed that there is no link between the presence of an abnormality such as a clinical sign and other clinical signs seen in that disease. Signs can be related in terms of pathophysiology, and will occur together more frequently than if conditionally independent. Conditional independence of signs is assumed because the sensitivities of the sets of clinical signs within diseases are largely unknown, or not reported. The frequency of occurrence of any combination of signs can be computed from the sign frequencies of the individual signs, if conditional independence is assumed.

### Prevalence

The use of a particular prevalence value when calculating probabilities may be inappropriate for a given individual exposed to unique risks. It is better to determine the risk factors operating on the animal in question at the time of the disease onset.

### Limitations in the use of diagnostic theory

Studies in human medicine have demonstrated a lack of ability to apply the probability theory objectively, even in the simplest applications. The human inability to perform the mathematical computations required and the availability of data are important limiting factors.

### Bayes' theorem with conditional independence

For a given disease, and a given finding (or set of findings):

Probability of disease =

$$\frac{\text{Probability of the finding in diseased animals} \times \text{Prevalence of the disease}}{\text{Probability of the finding being found in any animals in the population}}$$

or

$$P(D!S) = \frac{P(S!D) \times P(D)}{P(S)}$$

where:

$P(D!S)$ = the probability of the disease being present given that the particular sign (S) has been observed.
$P(S!D)$ = the probability of observing the sign (S) given that the disease is present.
$P(D)$ = the frequency of the disease in the population (the disease prevalence).
$P(S)$ = the frequency of the sign (S) in the population at large.

## 7.6.3 Pathophysiological reasoning (functional reasoning)

Using the clinical signs observed, the system and the lesion within the system is identified using knowledge of disease mechanisms (pathophysiology and anatomy). A differential list is then constructed using diseases which could explain the disease processes identified. An important clinical sign, in this context, is one that has an important role in the pathophysiology of the disease under consideration which may be responsible for many of the clinical manifestations of the disease, e.g. rumen pH in ruminal acidosis.

## 7.7   Which method of pattern recognition is used?

A study performed by one of the authors (Cockcroft 1998) included an investigation on the diagnostic methods used by different groups of clinicians. The conclusions of this study were:

- Veterinary students use pathophysiological reasoning most often
- Experienced veterinary surgeons use pattern matching most often
- Both groups use all three methods some of the time. Different methods may be used concurrently
- Pattern matching may be applied to diseases occurring in different prevalence bands.

## 7.8   Clinical reasoning strategies used in hypothetico-deductive reasoning

- The properties of clinical signs
- Logical exclusion of a disease
- Inductive and deductive reasoning
- Abstraction/aggregation
- Prevalence.

As the investigation proceeds, discriminatory information is collected in order to identify the location and cause of the disease. The process of interpreting the data is called clinical or diagnostic reasoning. It is this process that converts the database of information into a ranked list of most likely causes, and identifies the information required to confirm or rule out the competing hypotheses.

### 7.8.1   The properties of clinical signs

Clinical signs or combinations of clinical signs all have two properties for a given disease, the specificity and the sensitivity.

**Sensitivity** is the proportion of animals **with the disease with the sign**
**Specificity** is the proportion of the animals **without the disease that do not have the sign**.

The selection of a sign with a high sensitivity and specificity for a given disease can be used to confirm or rule out a diagnosis as the sign is likely to be present if the disease is present (high sensitivity) and does not occur in other diseases (high specificity). If the sign is absent the disease may be ruled out of further consideration.

The absence of a sign with a low sensitivity for a given disease does not rule in or rule out that disease and therefore conveys little additional information.

The presence of a sign with low specificity does not help differentiate the disease from other competing differential diagnoses.

For example, the detection of a 'ping' on from the left flank of a cow has both a high sensitivity and specificity for the diagnosis of a left displaced abomasum (LDA). Ketosis occurs in most cows with an LDA and also has a high sensitivity for an LDA. However, ketosis is present in several other diseases and is not exclusive to LDA. The specificity is therefore relatively low.

### 7.8.2   *Logical exclusion of a disease*

Diseases presenting clinical signs with sensitivities of either 0% or 100% can be eliminated from consideration if the signs are present or absent, respectively. Logical exclusion is a powerful strategy but may exclude the true diagnosis if the observation on which the exclusion is based is incorrect. Logical exclusion should be reserved for observations made with a high degree of certainty.

The presence of signs generally has a greater discriminatory power than the absence of signs. There are many more diseases with a particular sign absent (sign sensitivities = 0%) than diseases with it present (sign sensitivities > 0%). Thus a list of differentials based on the presence of signs will be shorter than one based solely on the absence of signs. However, considering both produces the shortest list.

### 7.8.3   *Inductive and deductive reasoning*

**Deductive** reasoning and **inductive** reasoning can be used alternately to investigate a hypothesis.

**Deductive reasoning**: If a cow is pale then the cow may have haemolytic anaemia.
**Inductive reasoning**: If the cow has haemolytic anaemia then the cow may have haemaglobinuria.

This method of reasoning can be used to test the strength of a hypothesis against competing hypotheses by identifying additional clinical signs to investigate.

### 7.8.4   *Abstraction/aggregation*

Abstraction is a way of summarising a group or complex of signs (in the same way that an abstract of a journal paper is a reduced version of the whole paper).

Abstraction is a useful way of grouping a number of conditionally dependent signs together to create a single pathophysiological process.

In cattle, a condition comprising tachycardia (increased heart rate), tachypnoea (increased breathing rate), cyanosis, submandibular oedema, and brisket oedema, could be abstracted to congestive heart failure. Similarly, pale mucous membranes, tachycardia, tachypnoea, low PCV, and recumbency, could be abstracted to anaemia.

By reducing the problem to a pathophysiological description only, diseases that produce that pathophysiology need to be considered.

### 7.8.5 Prevalence

'If you hear hoof beats think horses, unless you are in a zoo, then think zebras.'

The relative prevalences of competing differential diagnoses are important information in the diagnostic process. By using broad bands of different prevalence values it is possible to confine the initial search to diseases that are known to occur commonly.

The use of prevalence in probabilities represents a geographical average which may be inappropriate for a given individual, in a given environment. It is important to determine the risk factors operating on the animal in question at the time of the disease onset. For example, milk fever is a common condition in periparturient high yielding older cows but the prevalence amongst dairy cows in general is much less common.

## 7.9 Errors in hypothetico-deductive reasoning

Research on problem solving has demonstrated that human beings consistently make systematic errors. These include:

- The collection of extraneous information which does not lead to the confirmation or testing of a hypothesis
- Failure to retrieve the correct hypotheses from memory
- Data collection driven by an inappropriate hypothesis
- New data is generally considered only in relation to the hypothesis that is being tested and not in relation to alternative hypotheses
- Information that does not fit the differential diagnoses under consideration may be ignored in preference to generating alternative hypotheses
- Inexperienced clinicians tend to seek confirmatory information rather than rule out information reducing their diagnostic efficiency further.

The most common cause of incorrect diagnoses is a failure to generate, and therefore consider, the correct diagnostic hypothesis.

Saliency means a striking point or feature or highlight. Saliency bias occurs in diagnosis when a particular disease highlight, or presentation, makes it much easier to remember than other more common diseases. This is often influenced by a recent exposure to such a highlight, its unique clinical features, the rarity of a disease or the experience of having misdiagnosed a case in the past. Students tend to suffer from this as a result of receiving much of their teaching in referral centres. A bias is introduced which causes an overestimate of the probability of disease. For example, a recent case of chylothorax in a cat may bias the diagnostic work-up in the next few cases of cats presenting with dyspnoea.

## 7.10 Logic, sets, Venn diagrams, Boolean algebra

This section links this chapter and the next chapter. An understanding of data structures which can be used to represent disease will increase your understanding of your own clinical reasoning as well as that used by clinical diagnostic decision support systems which are described in the next chapter.

Clinical manifestations of disease can be represented using symbolic logic and set theory (figure 7.2). These enable deductive and inductive reasoning to be represented in the form of Venn diagrams and Boolean algebra. Venn diagrams

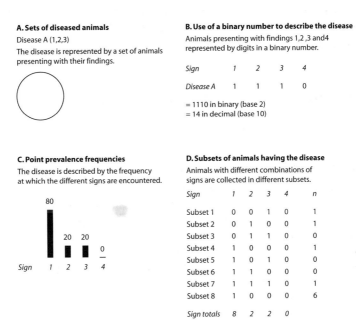

**Fig. 7.2(A–D)**  An illustration of four ways in which the signs of a disease can be represented mathematically

are able to depict the cluster of manifestations that form the clinical spectrum of a disease. Using these approaches sets of signs representing diseases can be expressed in binary form suitable for computerisation and Boolean algebraic operations (figure 7.2B).

### 7.10.1   Clinical sign sensitivities

Clinical sign sensitivities are the expected frequencies seen with a particular disease (figure 7.2C). The point prevalence frequencies are stage contact sensitive. If the time of observation is predominantly at a late stage in the course of a disease, the frequencies would be expected to be different from those seen at an earlier stage. Sign sensitivities do not indicate the conditional dependence of the clinical signs or the frequency of sign combinations.

### 7.10.2   Disease subsets

It is possible to identify subsets or clusters of clinical signs leading to different prognoses. The sign sensitivities can be subdivided into similar subsets (figure 7.2D). These subsets are the set frequencies required for conditional dependence in Bayes' theorem. They also represent different stages in the severity of the diseases. They can relate to prognosis, and may indicate the suitability of certain therapies.

The lack of information regarding disease clinical profiles has been identified as a limiting factor in veterinary diagnosis.

### 7.10.3   Venn diagrams and Boolean algebra

Venn diagrams and Boolean algebra can be used to describe the relationship between diseases with regard to their clinical signs in a formal way. An example using four conditions and three clinical signs is shown in figure 7.3.

*ntersection (∩), the logical AND*

This is represented by the overlapping area of the Venn diagram. A disease with the clinical signs red urine and jaundice and pale such as haemolytic anaemia can be presented mathematically as:

Red urine ∩ Jaundice ∩ Pale, or
Red urine AND Jaundice AND Pale.

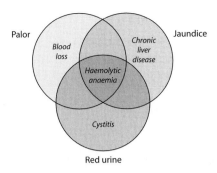

| | Palor | Jaundice | Red urine |
|---|---|---|---|
| *Blood Loss* | + | - | |
| *Chronic liver disease* | - | + | - |
| *Haemolytic anaemia* | + | + | + |
| *Cystitis* | - | - | + |

**Fig. 7.3** A Venn diagram showing the links between blood loss, chronic liver disease and cystitis, with the signs of palor, jaundice, and red urine

## Union (∪), the logical OR

This is represented by the combined areas of the circles in the Venn diagram. Diseases with the clinical sign red urine, or jaundice, or pale, can be presented mathematically as:

Red urine ∪ Jaundice ∪ Pale, or
Red urine OR Jaundice OR Pale.

## (⁻), the logical NOT

The complement of a set, i.e. animals excluding those contained in a set, is the area of the Venn diagram other than the area representing the set in question. Diseases that have jaundice, but not haemaglobinuria or palor, can be written as:

Jaundice ∩ $\overline{\text{(Haemaglobulinuria ∪ Pale)}}$, or
Jaundice AND NOT (Haemaglobulinuria OR Pale)

The full set of logical operators includes NAND (not and), NOR (not or), XOR (exclusive or), and XNOR (exclusive not or) which are compound operators. They are produced by combining the functions of the basic AND, OR and NOT operators.

## 7.11   Clinical staging of metritis in cattle

Clinical staging can be represented in the form of Venn diagrams and Boolean algebra and an example using metritis in cows is shown below. Three clinical signs are used to categorise the condition into mild, moderate or severe.

Patients can be categorised according to the severity of the disease by where they are placed in the Venn diagrams as illustrated in figure 7.4.

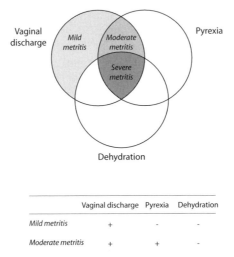

|  | Vaginal discharge | Pyrexia | Dehydration |
|---|---|---|---|
| *Mild metritis* | + | - | - |
| *Moderate metritis* | + | + | - |
| *Severe metritis* | + | + | + |

**Fig. 7.4**   An illustration of how the severity of bovine metritis can be represented using a Venn diagram

## References and further reading

Blood, D.C. and Brightling, P. (1988) *Veterinary Information Management*. Baillière-Tindall, London.

Campbell, E.J.M., Scadding, J.G. and Roberts, R.S. (1979) The concept of disease. *British Medical Journal* **2**, 757–62.

Cockcroft, P.D. (1996) Pattern matching models of veterinary diagnosis. DVM&S thesis, University of Edinburgh.

Cockcroft, P.D. (1998) A survey of pattern recognition methods in veterinary diagnosis. *Journal of Veterinary Education* **25** (2), 21–3.

Miller, R.A. and Geissbuhler, A. (1999) Clinical diagnostic decision support systems: an overview. In *Clinical Diagnostic Decision Support Systems* (ed. Berner, E.S.). Springer, New York, pp. 3–34.

Radostits, O.M., Tyler, J.W. and Mayhew, I.G.J. (2000) Making a diagnosis. In *Veterinary Clinical Examination and Diagnosis* (eds Radostits O.M., Mayhew, I.G.J. and Houston D.M.). W.B. Saunders, London, pp. 11–52.

Smith, R.D. (1995) *Veterinary Clinical Epidemiology*. Butterworth-Heinemann, London.

White, M.E (1988) Diagnosis, information management, and record coding using the Consultant database. *Canadian Veterinary Journal* **29**, 271–3.

# Review questions

Can you write down and draw out in the form of a flow diagram your next clinical work-up illustrating the process from the initial observations to the final diagnosis? Use the following questions to help you.

## *Clinical examination*

**1** *Which method of clinical examination did you use?*

(a)   Complete clinical examination
(b)   General clinical examination followed by hypothetico-deductive approach
(c)   General examination followed by a complete examination of system/topographical area.

## *Clinical reasoning*

**2** *When using the hypothetico-deductive (problem-orientated) method of clinical examination and clinical reasoning, did you follow the following steps?*

(1)   Collection of data (clinical examination, laboratory tests)
(2)   The recall of possible differential diagnoses (hypotheses)
(3)   Ranking of competing differential diagnoses
(4)   Further investigations to enable differentiation of the competing hypotheses
   • evidence strongly in favour of particular diagnosis, go to 5
   • still unable to decide on a diagnosis, go to 1
(5)   Diagnosis confirmed, closure.

**3** *When formulating a differential diagnosis list do you:*

(a)   Recall diseases which contain all the signs observed?
(b)   Recall diseases which contain only signs you are confident about?
(c)   Recall diseases for each sign?
(d)   Recall diseases which contain most of the signs observed?
(e)   Recall diseases which contain an important sign?
(f)   Recall only common diseases?

**4** *When ranking the differential diagnosis list, which method of pattern recognition did you use?*

(a)   Pattern matching
(b)   Probabilities
(c)   Pathophysiological reasoning.

**5** *Which of the following strategies did you use?*

    (a)   The specificities and sensitivities of clinical signs
    (b)   Logical exclusion of a disease
    (c)   Inductive and deductive reasoning
    (d)   Abstraction/aggregation.

**6** *Have you identified outstanding information needs such as:*

    (a)   Epidemiology of the disease
    (b)   Prevalence of disease
    (c)   Risk factors present or absent
    (d)   Pathophysiologies that may be present in the disease
    (e)   Signs present and absent in a disease
    (f)   The range and frequency of clinical case presentations in a disease
    (g)   The sensitivity and specificity of the signs and clinical case presentations
    (h)   The association between risk factors and the presence of the disease
    (i)   The prevalence of the disease in the population from which the animal came
    (j)   The time course of the disease
    (k)   Sample size to detect herd infections at a given prevalence of disease
    (l)   The true ranges of normal physiological parameters and what the likelihood is of disease in an animal with a given value
    (m)  Use of clinical decision support systems.

# 8

# CLINICAL DIAGNOSTIC DECISION SUPPORT SYSTEMS (CDDSSs)

The aim of this chapter is to introduce the theory behind the development of clinical diagnostic support systems (CDDSSs) and to provide some examples of veterinary systems.

On completion of this chapter readers should:

- Understand the methods used by CDDSSs
- Understand how the performance of such systems can be evaluated
- Have a basic knowledge of the mechanisms and operation of CDDSSs available to veterinary practitioners.

125

## 8.1   Introduction

It will be difficult for many readers to embark on this chapter with an open mind. Most of us have preconceptions on the subject of computer assisted problem solving. In the previous chapter we scratched the surface of the complexity involved in reaching a diagnosis, and it would be naïve in the extreme, to believe that decision support systems will play a major part in the daily work of a veterinary diagnostician in the foreseeable future. However, as a relatively unsophisticated tool (when compared with the human brain), they may have a useful role to play in particular clinical situations, and as an educational tool. They can provide reassurance that we haven't missed the obvious, and they can provide that extra piece of evidence that reduces uncertainty. Their development will continue, and whether readers view this with unease or with interest, there is no doubt that some understanding of the reasoning used to create CDDSSs, and an awareness of the knowledge used to drive them, will enable readers to arrive at an informed opinion on their potential role in veterinary medicine.

Past and present CDDSSs incorporate inexact models of the incompletely understood and exceptionally complex process of clinical diagnosis. However, it is best to conceive the process not as a single event, but as a series of different processes. CDDSSs are at their most powerful when they provide information about one aspect of the process and allowing the clinician to form a judgement. They are used to supplement the clinician's own diagnostic capabilities. There are often unrealistic expectations of their performance. The user needs to be aware and understand the assumptions built into the system.

Motivations to understand and to automate the process of clinical decision making have included a desire to improve the:

- accuracy of clinical diagnosis
- reliability of clinical decisions
- understanding of the structure of medical knowledge
- understanding of clinical decision making.

### 8.1.1   Definition

A CDDSS is a system that assists a clinician with one or more component steps of the diagnostic process. There are systems for general diagnosis, and for diagnosis within a specialised domain, such as the interpretation of laboratory data or blood gas analysis.

All CDDSSs should make their methodology, reasoning and sources of information explicit. In addition there should be a measure of their proficiency, such as accuracy, or ideally their specificity and sensitivity.

### 8.1.2 Questions you should ask

Because the published performance indices of expert systems are often difficult to interpret, or even absent, it is important that other aspects of the construction of the CDDSS are critically appraised.

(1)  What is the source of the clinical information within the system?

- Is it based on expert opinion?
- Is it derived from the literature?
- Is it derived from a database of cases?

(2)  Is the information derived from the same population as I wish to use the system for?

(3)  If disease clinical sign frequencies are used, is it likely that they are the same in my population? Remember, sign frequencies will be different depending on the stage of disease at which the veterinary surgeon is requested to examine the animal.

(4)  In addition to entering the signs I have observed, does the system enable me to enter signs I have not seen or signs I have not examined?

(5)  If prevalence is used, is it:

- Expert opinion derived?
- Obtained from cross-sectional surveys?
- The same in my population?
- The prevalence that is presented to the veterinary surgeon?
- The true prevalence of disease?

(6)  Do I understand how the expert system works?

(7)  What is the result telling me?

(8)  Does the expert system use a pattern recognition system based upon assumptions that may make the output inaccurate? For example, if the expert system uses probabilities to generate the probability of a disease using a given set of clinical signs, is conditional independence assumed?

(9)  If information is provided regarding the performance of the CDDSS, do I understand what it is telling me?

## 8.2 Understanding the methodology used by CDDSSs

Clinical information is rarely categorical. Signs within diseases are rarely present in 100% of encounters. Dealing with this uncertainty is a major challenge in designing more complex and useful CDDSSs. This section describes various methods that have been used in CDDSSs.

Pattern recognition techniques are an important component in medical decision support systems and are used for the classification of a patient into a diagnostic or treatment group. The pattern recognition methods used are:

- pathophysiological
- pattern matching
- probability.

The methods used to arrive at diagnoses in automated systems have included:

- logic (set theory, Venn diagrams and Boolean algebra)
- pattern matching
- probabilities with and without conditional independence (Bayes' theorem)
- knowledge-based systems using production (If . . . then rules) and relational syntactical networks with or without hierarchical and aggregation structures
- Bayesian belief systems
- neural networks.

### 8.2.1   Logic

Logic (as embodied in set theory and Boolean algebra) is an important and powerful concept in medical reasoning. For example, a disease can be excluded if a sign is observed which has never been recorded in the disease. This of course assumes that there is a single condition affecting the animal and that the recorded signs for a disease are complete and absolute. In spite of these criticisms, logic still remains the most dominant pattern recognition method in simple CDDSSs.

When considering differential diagnoses, books tend to list conditions by single sign, syndrome or simple pathophysiology. Books become less useful when considering different combinations of multiple signs. It is by considering the causes of the combinations of signs that we are able to narrow the possibilities down most rapidly. Before the use of digital computers became possible, mechanical devices such as punch-edged and feature cards were used for this purpose. Relational computer databases have now superseded these. Consultant, which is described below, is a veterinary CDDSS translating clinical signs into a list of diseases that manifest the set of signs entered.

With categorical information, i.e. a sign is present or not, simple algorithms consisting of a series of branching decision nodes can be devised. However, uncertainty regarding the information requested at a node results in the need for an additional branch labelled 'don't know' or 'no further progress can be made down the algorithm'. These systems work well if the algorithm is short and uses categorical information only, but they are weak with more complex diseases and domains with greater uncertainty. Medical decision making embodies uncertainty, and functional reasoning in addition to quantitative information is not easily accommodated by these systems.

Logical systems based on discriminating between exclusive alternatives have used production rules (If . . . then). However, production rules (If . . . then) do not deal effectively with uncertainty, which is a considerable disadvantage.

### 8.2.2 List matching

List matching compares a patient's disease profile with stored profiles of diseases in the database. PROVIDES and Consultant are two computer-based veterinary examples of list matching diagnostic algorithms.

Consultant requires the input of a clinical sign or signs. From this it generates the differential diagnoses, a list of diseases which produce the sign or signs. This is a simple list matching procedure.

PROVIDES generates a differential diagnosis list by comparing the patient's attributes with a profile of expected findings for each disease. The system creates a list of differential diagnoses by comparing patient characteristics with patterns of discriminatory findings ('propensities') for each disease. The profile consists of findings that are strongly associated with the disease and which at the same time tend to differentiate it from other potential causes of the patient's problems. Diseases are then ranked according to the ratio of findings exhibited by the patient to those expected for the disease.

PROVIDES does not attempt to arrive at a single diagnosis but rather is intended to provide a list of reasonable possibilities for the clinician to consider. No disease is excluded just because it cannot account for all of the patient's signs.

The most common of the matching procedures involves the assignment of a weight to each sign for each disease. The signs of the patient are then summed according to their weight for each disease. The disease yielding the largest ratio of the patient's weighted sum of signs, to the weighed sum of all the characteristics of that disease, is considered the correct diagnosis. This procedure is called weighted summation.

### 8.2.3 Probabilities (Bayes' rule)

Systems using conditional dependence have an almost infinite data requirement to create an effective system, therefore most current systems assume sign conditional independence.

Bayes' theorem, assuming condition independence of all the clinical signs, has been adopted widely in medical diagnostic decision support systems. Bovid is a cattle disease decision support system and is an example of this type of system. These systems depend on large amounts of data, which must include the prevalence and sign sensitivities of the diseases. Often this information is based upon expert opinion and not on field data.

The main problems are ensuring the accuracy of the information within the database, and the assumption of conditional independence, which is likely to be untrue as pathophysiological processes result in linked disease manifestations.

### 8.2.4 *Knowledge-based systems incorporating symbolic reasoning (syntactical systems)*

Knowledge-based systems are usually composed, at least in part, of production (If ... then) rules. Some examples of production rules are:

- If the animal is male, then it cannot be pregnant (categorical rules)
- If the cow has severe milk fever then she will be recumbent (cause to effect rules)
- If the cow is hypocalcaemic then the diagnosis is milk fever (effect to cause rules)
- If the scouring calves are at grass then consider parasitic gastroenteritis (association rules).

More commonly they are used in semantic networks or combined with frames. A semantic net consists of nodes linked by arcs. This structure explicitly describes the relationships between nodes. These structures can be used to represent the pathophysiological and anatomical relationships in a disease process. Diarrhoea and dehydration could be nodes linked by an arc, 'causes', producing 'Diarrhoea "causes" dehydration'. Complex relationships can be represented by cross-linking nodes. Using these networks, complex functional patterns can be simplified using aggregation or hierarchical decomposition thus simplifying the diagnostic process. For example, congestive heart failure may be derived from a collection of clinical signs and the causes of congestive heart failure will then be explored.

Hypothesis-directed reasoning has been used in human medicine CDDSSs and uses forward chaining and backward chaining (inductive and deductive reasoning). The clinician enters a list of pertinent patient attributes, e.g. signs which are absent or present. This initial dataset evokes a set of disease hypotheses that are partitioned into subsets of competitors using an algorithm. The set of the most highly supported hypotheses then become the focus of attention and the program enters a questioning mode in which manifestations are requested in accordance with their ability to help sort out the best hypothesis among the competing set. Scores are recalculated as the clinician enters the data and the focus may shift as hypotheses are rejected or confirmed by the new information. Bovid, which is described below, has an interrogation mode which uses this methodology.

### 8.2.5  Bayesian belief networks

Bayesian belief networks, also called probabilistic causal networks or Bayesian networks, represent a merger of symbolic or artificial intelligence and Bayesian probabilities. Belief systems make dependences explicit and use probability theory.

Bayesian belief networks provide a method for representing probabilistic dependences and independences. Relationships between observations, inter-mediate states, and diagnosis can be expressed on a continuum from full independence to full causal dependence.

Bayesian belief is the probability of the sign(s) (observation(s)) given that the disease is present. It does not rely on the probability of the disease being present given the sign(s) (observation(s)) which would need disease prevalence data. This distinction is important to understand. The Bayesian belief network operates by updating the posterior probabilities of all the diseases, as each observation is entered. The numbers which the Bayesian network generates are known as beliefs because they describe the belief which we might have in different diseases, given the observation of particular pieces of evidence (observations). We may have an estimate of our belief in whether a cow is infected with listeriosis, given that we have observed that it has facial nerve paralysis. If we now observe the animal to be pyrexic this will change our belief in whether it has the disease.

### 8.2.6  Neural networks

Neural networks are computer-based pattern recognition methods with archi-tectural similarities to the nervous system. Nothing is stored in a single location: all knowledge is implicit in the pattern of the system's interconnections.

Individual variables of the network, usually called neurones, can receive inhi-bitory or excitatory inputs from other neurones. The networks can define relationships among input data that are not apparent using other approaches and they can use these relationships to improve accuracy. Neural nets can recognise patterns in complex datasets. They can be dynamic and temporal showing state changes with time in response to external inputs. The connectivity of a neural network determines its structure. Patterns are identified by the output of the system. They can be used to combine uncertain information with gate-ways operating dependent upon a certain threshold being attained.

## 8.3  Sources of uncertainty or inaccuracies

All the artificial intelligence approaches use heuristic (estimated) measures for scoring the weight of confidence or credibility to a hypothesis. These are usually uncertainty values attached by human experts to the various reasoning rules in the model. A certainty factor for a rule represents the expert's confidence in it, but it is not always clear what 'confidence' means. Whatever the meaning, the effect of the certainty factor on a rule is to weight the belief in its conclusions: the higher the rule's certainty factor, the higher the belief in the conclusions from that rule. Certainty beliefs are represented by numbers. It is difficult to be clear what the certainty factor means, other than to say higher numbers mean stronger beliefs.

## 8.4   Evaluation of the performance of CDDSSs

It is important that the user has a clear indication of the performance of a CDDSS. However, the validation of CDDSSs has been less than ideal. Accuracy is commonly used as a parameter of performance. Below are some of the methods that have been used to indicate the performance accuracy of CDDSSs.

- Using a selection of literature case reports based on availability
- Using a number of cases which have subsequently been examined at post-mortem, and a 'Gold standard' diagnosis obtained within a hospital environment
- Using a number of cases for which a putative diagnosis is made
- Defined by a correct diagnosis being at the top, or in the top 5, of a list of ranked differential diagnoses
- By asking experts if the rank and probabilities produced seem to be realistic
- By measuring the impact of patient outcomes in case–control studies
- In different practice settings, and different geographical areas, to assess the impact on performance with different populations
- By comparing the system with the performance of clinicians at different experience levels when presented with the same information.

### 8.4.1   *Which is the best method to measure the performance of a CDDSS?*

The performance of a CDDSS is often defined in terms of accuracy when presented with a number of diagnostic problems to solve. However, this parameter only considers the performance in animals that have a disease, and ignores those that don't have a disease.

As with all diagnostic tests, the ideal parameters of performance are the sensitivity and specificity for each disease within the system, using representative case reports from the population for which the system was devised. Likelihood ratios for a given test result with confidence intervals could be defined and the probability of the correct result being correctly computed. This has been reported for a pattern matching CDDSS for the differential diagnosis of bovine spongiform encephalopathy in cattle (Cockcroft 1999). In a large database with many diseases it is unlikely that such information would be available with sufficiently small confidence intervals (i.e. tested on enough cases).

To reduce the information required, a random sample of the diseases within the database could be analysed. An alternative to using a sample of case reports representative of the population to define the specificity would be to use a case report of each disease in the database apart from the disease under evaluation. This assessment of performance would be independent of any population, but similarly would not then relate to a specific population, however it would standardise CDDSS performance evaluation.

### 8.4.2 *Alternative desirable indicators of performance using accuracy*

- The accuracy of the system when compared with the performance of clinicians at different experience levels when presented with the same information
- The use of cases which are representative of the user's target population
- Accuracy with narrow confidence intervals (large number of cases used).

## 8.5   Veterinary diagnostic decision support systems

Decision support systems within veterinary science have been developed in a wide range of domains. In spite of this, the uptake and usage is still low. CDDSSs have ranged from clinical pathology and ECG analytical and diagnostic software programs for dogs and cats (VetSoft) to herd-level diagnostic programs for mastitis in cattle (Hogeveen *et al.* 1995a, b). Listed in table 8.1 is a selection of systems illustrating the wide range of methods used. It is a cause for concern that the pattern recognition method used in the CDDSS is often not described in detail and the source of data used is often not stated. Validation of systems is frequently absent, inappropriate or inadequate.

Following are some examples to help the reader gain experience in understanding the methodology and critical appraisal of the systems.

### 8.5.1 *A decision support algorithm for individual cow infertility*

The clinical signs associated with infertility are often absolute or categorical, and it is possible to produce a branching algorithm which provides a diagnostic pathway. As with all categorical algorithms, progression down the branches is reliant upon a specific item of information being available.

The algorithm begins by classifying the patient into one of four categories:

- no signs of oestrus
- short oestrus intervals
- normal oestrus intervals
- prolonged oestrus intervals.

Having established that the problem is one of short oestrus intervals, the algorithm illustrated in figure 8.1 can be followed.

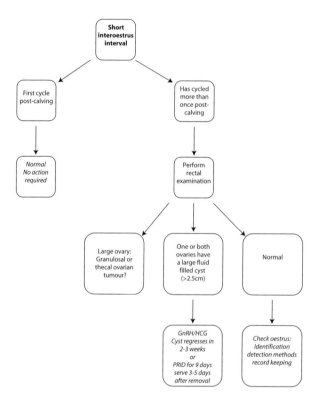

**Fig. 8.1**   An example of a diagnostic tree used to diagnose and treat the cause of a short interoestrus interval in a cow

## 8.5.2   Consultant

Consultant is a veterinary diagnostic support system used to suggest possible causes for clinical signs and to provide a brief synopsis of the cause including:

- a general description of the disease
- species affected
- the signs observed reported in the published literature
- a list of recent literature references.

**Table 8.1**  A list of some of the clinical diagnostic decision support systems which have been developed for veterinary science.

| System | Method used | Information source | Purpose | Source |
|---|---|---|---|---|
| 1. Cattle fertility (Noakes 1997) | Branching algorithm | Literature | Cattle fertility Diagnosis/ examination algorithm | Published literature |
| 2. Consultant (White 1988) | List matching | Literature | Differential diagnosis – all species | Online |
| 3. Canis (equus, felis) (Vetstream) | Branching algorithm | Expert opinion | Dog (horses and cats) diseases Examination and diagnosis | Subscription CD/online |
| 4. PROVIDES (Pollock and Fredericks 1988) | List matching | Literature | Examination and diagnosis | CD subscription |
| 5. Phytox (Animal Information Management) | Probability Conditional Independence | Literature and expert opinion | Diagnosis of plant poisoning | CD subscription |
| 6. Canid (Animal Information Management) | Probability Conditional Independence | Literature and expert opinion | Diagnosis of dog diseases | CD subscription |
| 7. Bovid (Animal Information Management) | Probability Conditional Independence | Literature and expert opinion | Diagnosis of cattle diseases | CD subscription |
| 8. Bovine spongiform encephalopathy (BSE) (Cockcroft 1999) | Pattern matching | Field cases | BSE differential diagnosis in cattle | Published literature |
| 9. EqWise | Weighting system Bayes' belief system | Expert opinion | Diagnosis of horse diseases | Online |
| 10. CaDDis (McKendrick *et al.* 2000) | Probability Bayes' belief system | Expert opinions | Cattle tropical diseases diagnosis | Online |
| 11. Biochemistry (Knox *et al.* 1997, 1998) | Probability | Hospital cases | Diagnosis in cattle and horses | Published literature |
| 12. Mastitis (Hogeveen *et al.* 1995a, b) | Knowledge-based (If … then) | Field | Diagnosis of mastitis at herd level in cattle | Published literature |

Dogs, cats, cattle, sheep, pigs, goats, birds and horses are the species represented.

The database consists of approximately:

- 500 signs
- 7000 conditions
- 18 000 literature references
- 3000 links to other websites where additional information can be obtained.

Consultant can be used by searching for information by diagnosis, and by searching of disease by sign(s).

In the search by diagnosis a search can be made for a particular condition using a key word. Matches to the key word are then displayed. Information regarding the nominated condition can then be obtained.

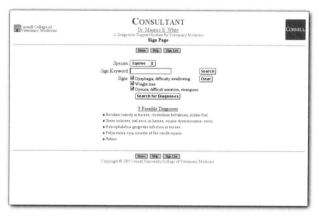

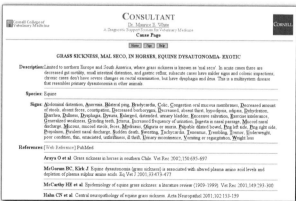

**Fig. 8.2**   Pages from the Consultant website illustrating the investigation of a case of grass sickness in a horse

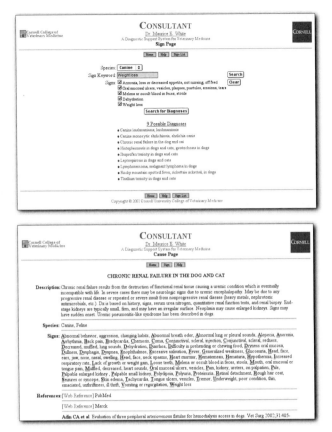

**Fig. 8.3** Pages from the Consultant website illustrating the investigation of a case of chronic renal failure in a dog

In the search by sign(s), a selection can be made of one or more signs in a nominated species and the search will then return all the diagnoses which contain all the signs (set of signs) which were entered. This represents a differential diagnosis list for the signs entered. The differential diagnoses are not ranked. It is important that the signs are entered accurately.

Two examples are used to illustrate Consultant. An equine case of grass sickness with signs of dysphasia, weight loss, and dysuria is entered. The results including the information available on grass sickness are shown in figure 8.2. A small animal case of chronic renal failure with the signs of anorexia, oral mucosal ulcers, melaena, dehydration, and weight loss is entered. The results including the information available on chronic renal failure in the dog are shown in figure 8.3.

### 8.5.3   *Vetstream Canis*

The Vetstream CD-ROMs are described briefly in Chapter 3. Within Canis there is a CDDSS called 'presenting problem'. A presenting syndrome such as poly-dypsia/polyuria or a sign is the starting point. The system takes the user through a series of questions for which a categorical answer is required such as absent/present, normal/abnormal. The system uses logic to retain or exclude conditions. The next question is designed to rule in or rule out diseases, producing a diminishing list of differential diagnoses. Retained differential diagnoses are categorised into likelihood bands. The likelihood bands reflect the incidences of the diseases, as all the clinical information collected is assumed to be absolute, and so no distinction is made other than the differences in incidence. All the information used is derived from expert opinion. No formal validation of the system using clinical data has been attempted. The algorithm can be drawn out as a branching tree with decision nodes for each question. An example of the system is shown in table 8.2 using an investigation of a dog with central diabetes insipidus. Help screens for each question provide the user with explanations or information related to the question that has been asked, and links provide more detailed information for performing tests or interpretations. Table 8.3 shows the list of differential diagnoses provided by Vetstream. This type of algorithm provides an audit trail of the decisions that have been made and provides strong evidence to defend the work-up.

### 8.5.4   *PROVIDES (Problem Orientated Veterinary Information and Decision System)*

PROVIDES uses a pattern-matching algorithm. It is a computer assisted diagnosis system for small animal medicine based upon the principles of the problem–knowledge coupler. Each item of information on the patient is coupled to relevant information from the literature. The system is modular, with each subunit covering a clinical sign or syndrome such as coughing or diarrhoea. The system obtains information by interrogating the user for information on signs, history, clinical and laboratory findings. The findings for a specific patient are compared to a representative profile of conditions in the computer using pattern matching. The computer then generates a ranked list of disease hypotheses based upon the proportion of the observed findings matching the expected findings (propensities). The propensities usually have a discriminatory value. For each disease this proportion is displayed. The condition with the highest proportion of matches is the most likely diagnosis. In addition the number of missing items of data which are represented in the database for each disease is highlighted. This is illustrated in table 8.4.

The information in the database is derived from the literature and is documented. The database also suggests tests to aid diagnoses, appropriate treat-

**Table 8.2**   Example of the questions and answers encountered during the investigation of central diabetes insipidus in a dog, using the Vetstream system.

| | | |
|---|---|---|
| Question 1 | Is the animal polydipsic and polyuric? | Yes |
| Question 2 | Is there a history of recent/current medication using any of the following?<br>Glucocorticoids<br>Mannitol<br>Dextrose<br>Diuretics<br>Phenytoin | No |
| Question 3 | If female, is she 2–8 weeks post-oestrus and showing signs of pyometra? | No |
| Question 4 | Have any of the following occurred:<br>Recent exposure to high temperatures?<br>Recent extreme physical exposure?<br>Recent change in diet to dry and salty food? | No |
| Question 5 | What are the urinalysis results<br>Glycosuria?<br>Proteinuria?<br>Normal? | Normal |
| Question 6 | What are the findings on routine biochemistry?<br>Decreased potassium<br>Increased urea and creatinine<br>Increased alkaline phosphatase | Normal<br>(Potassium = 4.0–5.5 mmol/l<br>Urea = 2.0–8.0 mmol/l<br>Alkaline phosphatase = 10–300 iu/l) |
| Question 7 | What are the results of the ACTH stimulation test or low dose dexamethasone suppression test?<br>Both test results normal<br>Both tests abnormal | Both test results normal |
| Question 8 | What is the urine specific gravity?<br>1.001–1.006<br>>1.007 | 1.001–1.006<br>(Normal range 1.015–1.040) |
| Question 9 | What is the result of the modified water deprivation test?<br>Water deprivation test concentrating urine (specific gravity > 1.025)<br>Water deprivation test does not result in increased concentration of urine | Unable to concentrate |
| Question 10 | How did the animal respond to anti-diuretic hormone?<br>ADH no response, no increase in urine specific gravity<br>ADH response, urine specific gravity > 1.025 | Concentrates urine in response to ADH |

**Table 8.3**  Example of the differential diagnoses considered during the investigation of central diabetes insipidus in a dog, using the Vetstream system.

| Differential diagnosis | Question leading to elimination |
|---|:---:|
| *Common* | |
| Chronic renal failure | 6 |
| Diabetes mellitus | 5 |
| Hyperadrenocorticism | 7 |
| Iatrogenic polydipsia | 2 |
| Pyometra | 3 |
| | |
| *Intermediate* | |
| Amyloidosis | 5 |
| Cystitis | 5 |
| Glomerulonephritis | 5 |
| Hepatic disease | 6 |
| Hypercalcaemia | 6 |
| Hypoadrenocorticism | 6 |
| Physiological causes of polydipsia | 4 |
| Pyelonephritis | 5 |
| | |
| *Rare* | |
| Acromegaly | 5 |
| Central diabetes insipidus | Not eliminated |
| Early renal failure | 8 |
| Fanconi syndrome | 5 |
| Hyperviscosity syndrome | 5 |
| Hypokalaemia | 6 |
| Nephrogenic diabetes insipidus | 9 |
| Post-acute renal failure | 6 |
| Primary renal failure | 5 |
| Primary renal glycosuria | 5 |
| Psychogenic polydipsia | 9 |

**Table 8.4**  Diseases A, D, C and D are ranked according to the number of matching clinical data points.

| Rank | Differential diagnosis | History obs/expected | Physical examination | Laboratory finding | Score | Missing data points |
|:---:|:---:|:---:|:---:|:---:|:---:|:---:|
| 1 | A | 2/2 | 2/2 | 1/1 | 5/5 | 3 |
| 2 | B | 2/2 | 2/2 | 2/3 | 6/7 | 2 |
| 3 | C | 1/1 | — | 2/3 | 4/6 | 1 |
| 4 | D | 0/1 | 1/1 | 1/2 | 2/4 | 3 |
| 5 | E | 0/1 | 1/1 | 0/2 | 1/4 | 3 |

ment, and possible outcomes for each disease together with literature references. The question and answer format is designed to prevent errors of omission that may occur when the clinician takes a history, and performs a clinical examination.

An example of the output from PROVIDES for a 10-year-old dog from the southwestern USA with a chronic, intermittent, productive cough, weight loss and lameness is shown in table 8.5. Radiographs and laboratory studies have not been completed, hence the large number of findings with no data.

**Table 8.5** Example of the output from PROVIDES for a 10-year-old dog from the southwestern USA with a chronic, intermittent, productive cough, weight loss and lameness.

| Rank | Cause | Present/expected | Missing data points |
|------|-------|------------------|---------------------|
| 1 | Heartworm | 3/4 | 5 |
| 2 | Chronic bronchitis | 3/4 | 0 |
| 3 | Coccidiodomycosis | 4/6 | 4 |
| 4 | Actinomycosis | 3/5 | 4 |
| 5 | General lymphosarcoma | 2/4 | 3 |
| 6 | Pulmonary neoplasia | 2/4 | 1 |
| 7 | Laryngitis | 2/4 | 0 |
| 8 | Lymphoid granulomatosis | 1/2 | 3 |
| 9 | Crenosoma vulpis infection | 1/2 | 0 |
| 10 | Tuberculosis | 3/7 | 1 |

Evaluation (Fessler 1984b).

Twenty cases of pruritis were studied prospectively. These cases were randomly selected. Entry of patient history and physical findings were made in a double-blind procedure. Entries were made without the knowledge of the clinician's differential diagnoses and the system's predictions were not made known to the clinician. Eleven cases of red eye (ocular inflammation) were similarly evaluated and 13 final diagnoses were made. The electrocardiogram interpreter included in PROVIDES was evaluated by selecting 10 animals, diagnosed from post-mortem examination, revealing 16 final diagnoses. In the pruritic dogs, the clinician defined 23 final diagnoses. Eighteen of the final diagnoses appeared in the first five rankings (78%). In the red eye dogs, all 13 final diagnoses appeared in the top five PROVIDES diagnoses for each case. In the ECG study of the 16 final diagnoses, PROVIDES placed 11 in the first five differentials.

## 8.5.5 Bovid

Bovid is an expert system for veterinary surgeons involved in the diagnosis, treatment and prevention of diseases of cattle. The database for Bovid-3 is compiled from the veterinary literature and the experience of a panel of senior veterinary clinicians and pathologists. There are 1044 different diseases in the database. For each disease, 1191 parameters are defined, including clinical pathology, haematology, pathological findings, gross pathology and histopathology. Each disease also has a summary of its aetiology, epidemiology, major risk factors, confirmatory tests, recommended treatments, control measures and cross-references to standard texts.

The diseases to be included in the database were compiled from standard textbooks and journals. The lists of signs, for each disease, were derived from *Veterinary Medicine* (Radostits *et al.* 1994) with additional signs being added by the authors when considered appropriate. The sign frequencies of each clinical sign for each disease is called the point prevalence frequency, and represents the likelihood of observing the signs during the first point of contact with the veterinary surgeon. In other words, they are the numbers of animals which would be observed with the signs, if presented with 100 cases of the disease. This quantitative data is very scarce in the veterinary literature, and so expert opinion was used to provide this data. Two, and sometimes three, veterinary surgeons were asked to provide a consensus view of the sign frequencies. The relative prevalence of each disease was estimated for the southern temperate region of Australia. The prevalence of each disease within the system can be configured to represent other populations.

**Table 8.6**   The initial signs that were entered for a case of enzootic haematuria and the questions asked and the answers entered for two interrogation cycles of the Bovid CDDSS.

| Initial signs entered | Interrogation 1 | | Interrogation 2 | |
|---|---|---|---|---|
| | Question | Answer | Question | Answer |
| Female | Calving, during first month afterwards | No | Feed intake < 50% of normal | No |
| Key signs | Lactating cow | No | Temperature > 39.5 | No |
| Adult | Patient number affected > 1 in outbreak | No | Blindness indicated by behaviour | No |
| Urine red | Course acute (complete > 24 h < 2 weeks | No | Cornea Opacity unspecified | No |
| Haematuria | Course recurrent attacks | No | Conjunctiva red/inflamed | No |
| | Mucosae haemorrhage | No | Eye discharge unspecified | No |
| | Urine cloudy | No | Eye discharge purulent | No |
| | Urine contains protein | No | Skin thick or wrinkled | No |
| | Urine contains pus | No | Skin hyperkeratotic | No |

**Table 8.7** The probabilities of differential diagnoses following the entry of the initial clinical signs, interrogation cycle 1 and interrogation cycle 2.

| Diagnosis | Probability | | |
|---|---|---|---|
| | Initial signs | Interrogation 1 | Interrogation 2 |
| Haematuria enzootic | 3 | 88 | 98 |
| Inherited thrombocytopathia | <1 | 1 | <1 |
| Pyelonephritis, contagious bovine | 36 | 1 | <1 |
| Pyelonephritis | 5 | <1 | <1 |
| Haematuria undifferentiated | 2 | <1 | <1 |
| Urinary bladder neoplasm | 1 | 1 | 1 |
| Cystitis | 52 | <1 | <1 |
| Inherited factor XI deficiency | <1 | <1 | <1 |
| Poisoning trichloroethylene extracted soyabean meal | <1 | <1 | <1 |
| Anaemia undifferentiated | <1 | 1 | <1 |
| Haemorrhagic disease undifferentiated | <1 | <1 | <1 |
| Inherited thrombopathy, dyskeratosis, progressive alopecia | <1 | 1 | <1 |
| Poisoning phosphorus | <1 | <1 | <1 |
| Bovine malignant cattarhal fever | <1 | 1 | <1 |
| Thrombocytopenia idiopoathic (immune mediated) | <1 | 1< | <1 |

**Table 8.8** Diseases which may present with melaena (faeces, black) and the sign frequencies for each disease.

| Disease | Sign frequency |
|---|---|
| Abomasal ulcer haemorrhagic type | 95% |
| Poisoning fossil oil | 95% |
| Poisoning sulphur | 95% |
| Abomasal ulcer perforating acute local peritonitis | 80% |
| Abomasal torsion | 70% |
| Intussception | 70% |
| Poisoning lead dumb form | 50% |
| Bovine viral leukosis alimentary form | 30% |
| Intestinal neoplasia | 30% |
| Abomasal rupture | 30% |
| Radiation injury | 30% |
| Abomasal perforating diffuse peritonitis | 20% |
| Intestinal obstruction acute | 5% |
| Lung abscessation | 5% |
| Vena caval caudal syndrome | 5% |
| Vena caval cranial syndrome | 5% |

This CDDSS uses Bayes' theorem assuming conditional independence of the signs. Probabilities are used to rank the likelihood of differential diagnoses. Signs are entered using a menu and the menus are arranged by body system. The sign can be recorded as either 'present' or 'absent'. Additionally, a sign recorded as 'present' can be further designated as a 'critical' or 'key sign'. These are important signs that the clinician is confident about. Diseases in which the sign doesn't occur are excluded. This enables uncertainty to be accommodated within the system as no disease is excluded from consideration unless it is excluded on the basis of a critical sign. When a small group of signs (a maximum of seven is suggested) is entered, with one marked as a key sign, a ranked list of differential diagnoses is produced with a probability attached to each disease listed. The algorithm follows a hypothetico-deductive approach in the search for additional information. The interrogation mode checks for the signs or lesions that would help to differentiate the diagnoses on the list. The system is not designed to handle cases of concurrent disease. An example using a case of enzootic haematuria is presented in table 8.6 and table 8.7.

The sign database enables lists of diseases to be generated for single signs, with the sign frequency for each disease listed, melaena is used as an example in table 8.8. Alternatively the disease database can be used to provide a list of the signs, and sign frequencies of those signs, occurring with a nominated disease. This is illustrated using wasting primary ketosis (acetonaemia) in table 8.9.

Evaluation and validation of the system has been attempted using 27 clinical

**Table 8.9** Signs frequencies for wasting primary ketosis (acetonaemia).

| Sign | Sign frequency |
|---|---|
| Female | 100% |
| Adult | 100% |
| Urine contain ketones | 100% |
| Lactating cow | 95% |
| Milk yield less than normal | 95% |
| Body weight less than normal | 95% |
| Faeces dry and firm | 95% |
| Hypoglycaemic | 95% |
| Calving, during first month | 70% |
| Hyporesponsive to external stimuli | 70% |
| Liver fatty on histology | 70% |
| Feed intake < 50% | 50% |
| Rumen rate slow (1–2/min) | 50% |
| Course > 2 weeks | 30% |
| Muzzle dry | 30% |
| Calving, immediately after | 5% |
| Dry cow | 5% |
| Pica | 5% |
| Heart rate < 70/min | 5% |
| Emaciated | 5% |
| Faeces scant and pasty | 5% |

cases from nine veterinary surgeons. In 23 out of 27 of the cases, the opinion of an independent senior veterinary surgeon was that the resultant lists were complete, and ranked correctly (Brightling *et al.* 1996).

### 8.5.6  *EqWise*

EqWise is an equine information system available on the Internet. Included in this site is a CCDDS containing modules for diarrhoea, lameness, coughing, skin problems, anaemia, heart murmurs, wasting, and the sick foal. Each category of disease provides a potential but incomplete list of diseases that may exhibit the problem category. The user is then taken through a list of questions pertinent to the remaining conditions. Diseases that never manifest the characteristic reported by the user are excluded. An example using the diarrhoea module to investigate an outbreak of salmonellosis in a group of horses is shown in figure 8.4. After each question has been answered, the remaining diseases are ranked according to the probability of the sign(s) given that the disease is present. There are links to further information for each disease.

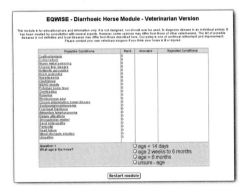

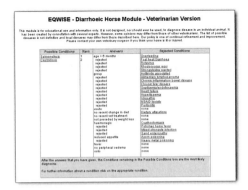

**Fig. 8.4**  Pages from the EqWise website illustrating the investigation of a case of salmonellosis in a group of foals

### 8.5.7　Cattle Disease Diagnostic System (CaDDiS)

This system uses a Bayesian belief network to aid differential diagnosis of tropical bovine diseases and is available via the Internet (figure 8.5). Information about 27 sign frequencies for 20 diseases were obtained by consulting 44 experienced

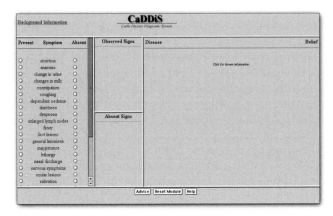

**Fig. 8.5**　A page from the CaDDis website

**Table 8.10**　The input and output using the CaDDis system.

| Present | Signs | Absent | Signs present | Diagnoses | Beliefs |
|---|---|---|---|---|---|
| | Abortion | | Anaemia | Babesiosis | 0.493 |
| + | Anaemia | | nervous signs | Chronic trypanosomiasis | 0.184 |
| | Change in urine | | | Facioliasis | 0.164 |
| | Change in milk | | | Acute trypanosomiasis | 0.149 |
| | Constipation | | | East coast fever | 0.010 |
| − | Coughing | | | | |
| | Dependent oedema | | | | |
| | Diarrhoea | | | | |
| | Dyspnoea | | | | |
| | Enlarged lymph nodes | | | | |
| | Fever | | | | |
| | Foot lesions | | Signs absent | | |
| | General lameness | | Coughing | | |
| | Inappetence | | | | |
| | Lethargy | | | | |
| | Nasal discharge | | | | |
| | Ocular lesions | | | | |
| + | Nervous signs | | | | |
| | Salivation | | | | |
| | Skin lesions | | | | |
| | Subcutaneous lesions | | | | |
| | Sudden death | | | | |
| | Sudden milk drop | | | | |

veterinary surgeons. The experts were asked to give opinions for those diseases of which they had experience. The method used within CaDDis is based on Bayes' theorem assuming the conditional independence of the signs within the disease. Prevalence of disease is not used. The result is the probability of the sign(s) given that the disease is present and not the probability of the disease being present given the sign(s) which would need disease prevalence data. This distinction is important to understand. There are definitions of the signs and more detailed information on the diseases if required. The system is based upon expert opinion and has not been validated. An example entering the signs anaemia present, nervous signs present and cough absent is presented in table 8.10.

### 8.5.8 *Application of probability techniques to the objective interpretation of veterinary clinical biochemical data*

This analysis was presented for a veterinary hospital population of horses (Knox *et al.* 1998) and cattle (Knox *et al.* 1997).

The usual method of interpreting clinical biochemistry results for an unwell animal is to compare the result with a reference range derived from healthy animals of the appropriate species, and if possible a similar age. It is then determined if the value lies within the normal range, or is outside it. If it is outside the range, the animal may be categorised according to the severity of the suspected underlying pathophysiology. Most normal ranges assume that the data is normally distributed, and ranges may represent a statistical band to include 95% of the normal population based upon this assumption.

By measuring biochemical parameters for a population of unhealthy animals, from a population appropriate to the patient, additional diagnostic information may be obtained from the parameter measured.

For a given population of unhealthy animals, each parameter measured is split up into percentile bands. For example, a percentile band of 6–10% for urea would exclude the lowest 5% and the highest 90% of urea values. This percentile band can be expressed as range of urea values. The diagnoses of the animals in the unhealthy population are known. The proportion of the population represented by each disease is known. The number of animals with each disease falling into the different percentile band is also known. From this information the following can be determined:

- *Pre-test odds*: the odds or probability of a disease being the cause of the unhealthy animal before the test
- *Post-test odds*: the odds or probability of a disease being the cause of the poor health in the animal after the test
- *Biochemical factor*: the effect that the new biochemistry value has on how many more times more likely a particular diagnosis is, given that the value lies in a particular percentile band.

For example, using a hospital database for horses, when the urea value lay in the lowest 5% of cases, hepatopathy had a biochemical factor of 3 indicating this result increased the pre-test odds by a factor of 3. However, when the urea value lay in the lowest 1%, the pre-test odds increased by a factor of 16 (table 8.11). In bovine cases a urea value of 30 mmol/l lay in the top 5% of all hospital case results and increased the pre-test odds of the disease being pyelonephritis by a factor of 8. A urea value that placed the cow in the top 1% of urea values increased the likelihood of a diagnosis of pyelonephritis by a factor of 16 (table 8.12).

**Table 8.11**   Biochemical factors for the diseases within selected percentiles of plasma urea in horses (Knox *et al.* 1998).

| Percentile | Urea mmol/l | Diagnosis | Biochemical factor |
|---|---|---|---|
| 1 (minimum) | 1.5–2.4 | Hepatopathy | 16 |
| 2–5 | 2.5–2.9 | Medical colic | 2 |
| | | Tooth root abscess | 6 |
| | | Colitis | 6 |
| | | Hepatopathy | 3 |
| | | Laminitis | 3 |
| 96–98 | 9.5–30.2 | Medical colic | 2 |
| | | Grass sickness | 6 |
| | | Hyperlipaemia | 12 |
| | | Surgical colic | 3 |
| | | Colitis | 6 |
| 99 (maximum) | 30.3–61.1 | Nephropathy | 34 |

**Table 8.12**   Biochemical factors for the diseases within selected percentiles of plasma urea in cattle (Knox *et al.* 1997).

| Percentile | Urea mmol/l | Diagnosis | Biochemical factor |
|---|---|---|---|
| 1 (minimum) | 0.870–1.051 | Chronic supparative pulmonary disease | 4 |
| 2–5 | 1.051–1.440 | Chronic supparative pulmonary disease | 2 |
| 96–98 | 29.314–55.343 | Ostertagiasis | 5 |
| | | Posterior vena cava syndrome | 3 |
| | | GI ulceration | 3 |
| | | Mucosal disease | 5 |
| | | Pyelonephritis | 8 |
| | | Johnes' disease | 3 |
| | | Ruptured bladder | 27 |
| 99 (maximum) | 55.344–120.000 | Nephropathy | 72 |
| | | Pyelonephritis | 16 |

This analysis therefore enables the probability of a disease to be determined given a biochemical value and identifies the most useful biochemical parameter, should a particular disease be suspected for a defined population.

The approach could equally be applied to all species in the general population.

## 8.6    Sources of information of the CDDSSs described in this chapter

### Biochemistry CDDSS

Knox, K.M.G., Reid, S.W.J., Irwin T., Murray, M. and Gettinby, G. (1997) Objective interpretation of bovine clinical biochemistry data: application of Bayes' law to a database model. *Preventive Veterinary Medicine* **33**, 147–58.

Knox, K.M.G., Reid, S.W.J., Love S., Murray, M. and Gettinby, G. (1998) Application of probability techniques to the objective interpretation of veterinary clinical biochemical data. *Veterinary Record* **142**, 323–7.

### Bovid, Canid and Phytox

These are commercial products available for purchase.

Animal Information Management, 209 Watton Street, Werribee, Victoria, Australia.

Brightling, P., Larcombe, M.T., Blood, D.C. and Kennedy, P.C. (1996) Development and the use of Bovid- 3, an expert system for veterinarians involved in diagnosis, treatment and prevention of diseases of cattle. *XIX World Buitrics Congress Proceedings* **2**, 528–32.

Radostits, O.M., Blood, D.C. and Gay, C.C. (1994) *Veterinary Medicine* 8th edition. Baillière Tindall, London.

### Bovine spongiform encephalopathy (BSE) CDDSS

Cockcroft, P.D. (1999) Pattern-matching models for the differential diagnosis of bovine spongiform encephalopathy. *Veterinary Record* **144**, 607–10.

### CaDDis

This program is available free of charge on the Internet at: http://vie.dis.strath.ac.uk/vie/CaDDiS/docs/Home_Page.html

McKendrick, I.J., Gettinby, G., Gu, Y., Reid, S.W.J. and Revie, C.W. (2000) Using a Bayensian belief network to aid differential diagnosis of tropical bovine diseases. *Preventive Veterinary Medicine* **47**, 141–56.

### Cardio and Hemo

This software is commercially available from VetSoft and further information and a demonstration can be found on the Internet at: http://www.dcn.davis.ca.us/~vetsoft/default.htm.

## Cattle fertility CDDSS

This algorithm was devised from:

Noakes, D.E. (1997) Fertility and infertility in the cow. In *Fertility and Obstetrics in Cattle.* Blackwell Science, Oxford.

## Consultant

Consultant is available on the World Wide Web at http://www.vet.cornell.edu

White, M.E. (1984) Consultant: computer-assisted differential diagnosis. *Veterinary Computing* **2**, 9–12.

White, E.W. (1988) Diagnosis, information management, teaching, and record coding using the consultant database. *Canadian Veterinary Journal* **29**, 271–3.

## EqWise

This program is available on the Internet. One demonstration module is free with a small registration fee to access the other modules. http://eqwise.gla.ac.uk

## Mastitis problems at herd level CDDSS

Hogeveen, H., Noordhuizen-Stazzen, E.N., Tepp, D.M., Kremer, W.D. and van Vleit, J.H. (1995a) A knowledge based system for the diagnosis of mastitis problems at the herd level. 1. Concepts. *Journal of Dairy Science* **78** (7), 1430–40.

Hogeveen, H., van Vleit, J.H. Noordhuizen-Stazzen, E.N., de Konning, C. Tepp, D.M., Brand, A. and Kremer, W.D. (1995b) A knowledge based system for the diagnosis of mastitis problems at the herd level. 2. Concepts. *Journal of Dairy Science* **78** (7), 1441–55.

## PROVIDES

These modular systems were commercially available some time ago but the authors have been unable to locate a source. Interested readers are directed to contact R.V.H. Pollock, Centre for Study of Medical Informatics, New York State College of Veterinary Medicine, Cornell University, Ithaca, NY 14853, USA.

Pollock, R.V.H. (1984) Provides: a veterinary information system. *Veterinary Computing* **2**, 4–8.

Pollock, R.V.H. (1985a) Anatomy of a diagnosis. *Compendium of Continuing Education* **7**, 621–30.

Pollock, R.H.V. (1985b) Diagnosis by calculation. *Compendium of Continuing Education* **7**, 1019–34.

Pollock, R.V.H. and Fredricks, T.A. (1988) Provides: a complete veterinary medical information system. *Canadian Veterinary Journal* **29**, 265–70.

## Vetstream Canis, Equus, Felis and Lapis

These are commercial products and can be obtained from: Vetstream Ltd, Three Hills Farm, Bartlow, Cambridge, CB1 6EN, UK; www.vetstream.com

# Further reading

Berner, E.G. (editor) (1998) *Clinical Decision Support Systems.* Springer-Verlag New York Inc.

Fessler, A.P. (1984a) Computer assisted decision-making in veterinary practice – 1. *Veterinary Medicine* **79**, 409–16.

Fessler, A.P. (1984b) Computer assisted decision-making in veterinary practice – 2. *Veterinary Medicine* **79**, 558–64.

## Review questions

Select the best answer to the following questions. Answers on page 205

**1** *Assuming conditional independence of clinical signs means:*

    (a)  Signs are considered to occur independently of one another
    (b)  The occurrence of signs is linked
    (c)  Sign frequencies cannot be multiplied together to compute the frequencies of combinations of signs
    (d)  The frequency of occurrence of combinations of clinical signs is accurate
    (e)  None of the above.

**2** *Taking into account conditional dependency means that:*

    (a)  Signs are considered to occur independently of one another
    (b)  The occurrence of signs is linked
    (c)  Sign frequencies cannot be multiplied together to compute the frequencies of combinations of signs
    (d)  The frequency of occurrence of combinations of clinical signs is accurate
    (e)  None of the above.

**3** *The best measure(s) of how good or bad a CDDSS is (are):*

    (a)  The accuracy
    (b)  The change in patient outcomes following the adoption of a CDDSS
    (c)  The specificity and the sensitivity
    (d)  The likelihood ratio(s) of a positive test and a negative test
    (e)  The level of agreement with experts.

**4** *Sign frequency (point prevalence frequency) is:*

    (a)  The proportion of animals with the disease which have the sign when presented to the veterinary surgeon for examination
    (b)  The proportion of animals which have the sign during the course of the disease
    (c)  The frequency with which the sign has been reported in the literature for that disease.

**5** *Information to be used in a CDDSS is best derived from:*

    (a)  Expert opinion
    (b)  Field cases
    (c)  Field cases from a comparative population for which the CDDSS is intended.

**6** *Ideally a CDDSS would take into account:*

(a) Disease prevalence
(b) Strongly associated disease risk factors
(c) Signalment
(d) Signs observed
(e) Signs not observed
(f) Signs not examined
(g) All of the above.

**7** *When evaluating a CDDSS the test data should consist of:*

(a) Cases used to construct the CDDSS
(b) Cases from a range of diseases represented in the database
(c) Cases from a range of diseases found in the target population.

**8** *Ideally, a CDDSS should be compared to:*

(a) Other CDDSSs
(b) Experts
(c) Undergraduates
(d) Newly qualified veterinary surgeons
(e) All of the above.

**9** *CDDSSs are most useful when used by:*

(a) Experts
(b) Non-experts.

**10** *Algorithms with decision nodes are best suited to:*

(a) Categorical clinical information
(b) Signs frequencies of 1–99%
(c) Simple categorical information for which answers to all the nodes are easily and quickly available.

*9*

# DECISION ANALYSIS, MODELS AND ECONOMICS AS EVIDENCE

The aim of this chapter is to provide an introduction to the use of decision analysis, economic factors, and the use of mathematical modelling as sources of evidence in the practice of evidence-based veterinary medicine.

After reading this chapter you should understand and be able to:

- Recognise appropriate situations in which decision analysis could be applied to decision making in veterinary practice and be able to carry out such a process
- Be able to incorporate financial factors into the decision making process
- Be able to calculate testing and treating thresholds
- Understand the methods used to create mathematical models of disease.

## 9.1   Introduction

It may seem to some readers excessively introspective to examine how we arrive at decisions, either at the general level or at a more specific level. In veterinary medicine we deal with greater uncertainty and with poorer levels of evidence than our medical counterparts. It sometimes feels as if we can divide the decision making into two categories: 'the self-evident' and 'it's anyone's guess'. There are times, however, when following an explicit decision-making process, when being more methodical enables us to be more confident in the conclusion, and certainly enables us to communicate more effectively with well-informed clients and colleagues when attempting to arrive at a consensus. When we use a methodical approach we can also include the owners' or clients' weighting on particular outcomes. These weightings are considered as utilities. For example, the owners of an old family pony will put a lower utility on return to full soundness, than the owner of a 2-year-old Thoroughbred in training, as an outcome of a lameness condition.

In large animal medicine, particularly when dealing with problems at the herd level, the use of models and the factoring of economic factors are powerful tools to help practitioners make decisions in our client's, and their animals', best interests.

This chapter goes into more detail than readers might expect in describing some aspects of mathematical modelling of infectious disease. We believe that a basic understanding of the methods used to produce the evidence that is used to formulate national policy is essential for those veterinary surgeons called upon to comment on or implement that policy.

## 9.2   Decision analysis

Decision analysis is the application of explicit quantitative methods to analyse decisions under conditions of uncertainty. When you are presented with a clinical problem with a number of options it is wise to ask the following question:

> 'Will the use of decision analysis identify the best course of action for the owner of my patient when two or more competing options exist?' (Friedland *et al.* 1998)

### 9.2.1   *Methods for clinical decision making*

- Dogmatism: This is the best way to do it
- Policy: This is the way we do it around here
- Experience: This way worked the last few times

- Whim: This way might work
- Nihilism: It doesn't really matter what we do
- Rule of least worst: Do what you will regret the least
- Defer to experts: How would you do it?
- Defer to patient: How would you like to proceed?

Optimal decision making requires veterinary surgeons to identify all possible strategies, accurately predict the probability of future events, and balance the risks and benefits of each possible action in consultation with the client. Decision analysis is a formalisation of the decision-making process. The decision tree is a flow diagram that outlines the outcomes that could follow each potential decision and calculates the probability and value of each event.

### 9.2.2　*Situations in which decision analysis may be helpful*

- A condition that has multiple competing treatment options with risks and benefits
- When important information may be missing. Decision analysis may identify critical information needs. This may be corrected by a literature search or following a search the uncertainty may still exist and this can be factored into the decision by using a wide range of reasonable subjective estimates
- When the owner's impact on the utilities is high
- When the risks may occur at different time points and the impact of this needs to be explained to the owner.

The method is explicit and quantitative. It forces the veterinary surgeon to consider all the options and outcomes. The product is the best option.

### 9.2.3　*The five steps in decision analysis*

(1)　Formulate an explicit question. Example: is T × A or T × B the best option?
(2)　Structure the decision and make the tree.
(3)　Obtain the data (probabilities and outcomes). Sources may include:
- *Clinical studies.* Studies reported in the literature provide the most reliable evidence as the data is quantitative and the literature peer reviewed. However, the population reported may not reflect the patient's population. It is important to ensure that the published probability applies to the patient's clinical situation.
- *Clinical database.* Local patterns of disease and outcomes of treatment may be more relevant than published data.
- *Expert opinion and educated guesses.* The accuracy of the subjective estimate is often dependent upon the experience of the individual. Several estimates are better than one.

(4)   Determine the value of each competing strategy.
(5)   Perform a sensitivity analysis for uncertain variables by using a range of values for the variables.

### 9.2.4   *Disadvantages of decision analysis*

The method is time consuming and laborious. However, once a tree is made it can be adapted for other patients with similar conditions. Computer programs are available to compute and draw the tree.

Decision analysis cannot be performed in the absence of evidence. Going through the 5-step approach will at least identify what information and level of evidence is available. This quantifies the uncertainty. Deconstructing a complex situation into component parts will help to identify the options.

Owner utilities may be unrealistic. Judgement is required to guide the owner through the process.

## 9.3   Decision trees

Decisions can be complex with many potential outcomes. While our brains are very good at rapidly processing many forms of complex information, we have a limited capacity to objectively interpret competing strategies with sufficient accuracy and reliability. Decision analysis provides a methodology to quantify the outcomes of decisions so that the best-informed choice, based upon the best external evidence and the owner's preferred values, can be identified. An appropriate and valid decision tree is the best technique for evidence-based decision making. It recognises the owner's value system, it can be quantitatively analysed and makes the clinical reasoning behind a decision explicit. An audit trail of clinical reasoning is produced. An example of a decision tree is shown in figure 9.1.

Decision trees are composed of:

- *Decision nodes.* Decision nodes indicate a conscious decision between two or more options. They are often depicted as squares in diagrams of decision trees.
- *Chance nodes.* No decisions are made at a chance node but likelihoods are attached to each outcome derived from the chance node. The likelihoods or probabilities of the outcomes emanating from a chance node add up to 1.0 or 100%, respectively. They are often depicted as circles in diagrams of decision trees.
- *Terminal nodes.* Terminal nodes are often represented as triangles or squares when no more decisions are taken. Utilities are attached to these terminal nodes to indicate the value attached to the outcome by the owner.

### 9.3.1   Utilities

Utilities use a 0–1 scale which reflects how important the outcome is to the owner. They are subjective in character. The best utility is given a value of 1.0 and the worst utility a value of 0.0. Every other outcome receives an intermediate score reflecting its relative value to the owner when compared to the two extremes. Utility scores do not have to add up to a specific number. These values should be rational and consistent. The utility then has to be multiplied by the probability of the outcome for which it has been defined to produce the expected utility. The expected utility with the highest value is the best option.

Deciding on utilities in veterinary medicine can be difficult as the animal's welfare must be safeguarded at all costs. However, it is important that the owner is able to express a preference. The choice of a utility is likely to be a consensus between veterinary surgeon and owner.

### 9.3.2   Solving the decision tree

In order to identify the outcome with the highest expected utility the probability of the terminal outcome has to be computed. This is accomplished by identifying each probability on the pathway from the terminal node to the root of the tree. These probabilities multiplied together give the probability of the outcome. If all the probabilities of the terminal nodes are added together they should come to 1.0 if likelihoods have been used, or 100% if probabilities have been used. This is a useful check on mathematical accuracy. The probability of the outcome is then multiplied by the utility to compute the expected utility.

Outcomes in many cases are still a matter of chance and it is important that the owner understands that the outcome with the highest expected utility may not be achieved.

### 9.3.3   Sensitivity analysis

Sensitivity analysis is performed to establish the relative importance of particular variables. If a variable is changed, how much does it have to be changed to make a significant difference to the outcome? One-way sensitivity analysis is when the value of one variable is changed. Two- and three-way sensitivity analysis is when two and three variable values are changed simultaneously. When we use estimated values (e.g. an estimated prevalence), sensitivity analysis is a good way of working out how accurate those estimates need to be.

### 9.3.4   Missing options

It is extremely important that options are not inadvertently omitted from the decision tree, as this will have an impact on the terminal outcome probabilities.

### 9.3.5   *Helping owners decide*

Decision trees are effectively mathematical models that enable us to look at the final outcome arising from a particular decision (or set of decisions). The construction of a decision tree requires detailed information on the probabilities of the various outcomes and the utility of the outcome to the patient. A utility is a value that is placed upon the outcome by the owner. That value may not be simply economic but may include the quality of life for the animal. The expected utility for each branch of the decision tree can be calculated from the probability of the outcome and the utility of the outcome. By examining the utilities of each terminal branch of the decision tree the best option can be identified to optimise the patient's welfare and/or the owner's wishes.

The construction of a decision tree and the decision analysis proceed in the following steps:

(1)   The tree is composed of clinical decisions for which all the relevant outcomes are defined.
(2)   A probability is attached to each of the outcomes for the decision.
(3)   The probability of the terminal outcome is the product of the probabilities of the preceding outcomes.
(4)   A utility is attached to the terminal outcome.
(5)   The option with the highest expected utility is selected.
(6)   The effect of changing any estimated probabilities and utilities can be assessed by changing their values and observing the effect on outcome values (sensitivity analysis).

Once the tree has been constructed check that:

- All the important treatment options and outcomes of these options (good and bad) are included in the construction of the tree
- The probabilities attached to the outcomes are based upon the best evidence and that they are credible
- The utilities are credible
- If estimates were used, were outcome utilities generated for a credible range of values?

The quality of the decision will only be as good as the estimates of the outcome probabilities and the outcome utilities. It provides patients with options that have been quantified. It also makes explicit the possible unfavourable outcomes.

Traditionally, much clinical decision making unconsciously follows the form of a decision tree but is not made explicit. By producing a decision tree it is possible to identify:

- All the potential outcomes of decisions
- The patient utilities or priorities of the animal and owner
- The gaps in the data required to complete the tree.

Economic decisions are frequently made by veterinary surgeons and their clients. The process of selecting a management plan involves an assessment of the available options and the probable outcomes. Decision analysis provides a framework for handling complex decisions so that they can be more objectively evaluated. A decision tree consists of nodes, which describe decisions, chances and outcomes. The tree is used to illustrate the strategies available to the veterinary surgeon and the likelihood of each outcome if a particular decision is made. Objective estimates of the outcomes may be derived from published research studies, records or subjective estimates.

### 9.3.6   *Obtaining utility values from clients and owners*

Utilities represent an owner's quantitative measure for a particular outcome. The utilities that are assigned to each of the outcomes are very subjective. They are not entities that we think of in numerical terms and so various techniques have been developed to aid their generation.

- Visual analogue scales
- Time trade-off
- Standard gamble.

*Visual analogue scales*

Visual analogue scales have been used to assist the owner. A visual analogue scale is a scaled line presenting a range of utility values for a given outcome, such as mild lameness in a dog following a given surgical procedure. It is found that humans tend to avoid placing a mark at the extremes of the scales and thereby introduce a bias.

*Time trade-off*

The owner is presented with a trade-off between the quality of life of the patient and the length of life left in time of the patient.

Consider the two health states, perfectly healthy and an impaired health status. Assume:

Time (*healthy*) × Utility (*healthy*) = Time (*impaired*) × Utility (*impaired*)

Time trade establishes that 4 years lived with a utility of 0.5 is equivalent to 2 years with a perfect utility of 1.0.

By getting the owner to choose relative time equivalences we are able to obtain the utility value.

If the patient was faced with a potential lifetime of 4 years with a severe limp, what reduction of lifetime would you be willing to accept for the dog to have perfect health? Let us assume that the owner says a reduction of 1 year (i.e. 3 years without a limp is equivalent to 4 years with a limp).

$$4 - 1 \ (healthy \ time) \times 1 \ (healthy \ utility) = 4 \ (impaired \ time) \times (impaired \ utility)$$

$$(impaired \ utility) = \frac{(4-1)}{4} = \frac{3}{4} = 0.75$$

The utility value calculated from the owner's views on the severe limp is 0.75.

### Standard gamble

In this scenario the owner is forced to choose between accepting a certain health state for the animal, or taking a gamble on a better outcome while risking the worst outcome.

The owner is presented with two doors. Behind door 1 is the certain outcome for an intermediate health state for which the utility is required from the patient. Behind door 2 are two hypothetical outcomes, the best possible outcome (complete recovery) or the worst possible outcome (death). The owner has to select which door to choose. By changing the probabilities of the two outcomes behind door 2 it is possible to reach a point where the owner finds it difficult to make a choice between door 1 and door 2. At this point the utility is equal to the probability of the best outcome behind door 2.

For example, most of us would open the second door if the likelihood of complete cure was 99.9%, and most of us would not open the second door if there were a 90% chance of death.

### 9.3.7 Decision analysis tree for therapeutic decisions

Figure 9.1 illustrates a decision tree for a condition that has a surgical and a medical option. In this example successful surgery with no pain or deformity is the best utility (1.0) and an outcome with pain and deformity is the worst utility (0.0). Multiplying the probability of each outcome with the utility of each outcome produces the expected utility for each outcome. Adding all the medical outcomes' expected utilities together gives the expected utility of the medical option, in this instance 0.525. Adding all the surgical outcomes' expected utilities together gives the expected utility of the surgical option, in this instance 0.830. The conclusion is that the outcome of the surgical option is likely to be better.

### 9.3.8 Decision analysis tree for economic decisions

Figure 9.2 illustrates a hypothetical economic decision analysis tree for three alternative therapies for treating mastitis in dairy cows when a recovery is inevitable. In this example the cost of a successful recover using treatment (Tx)

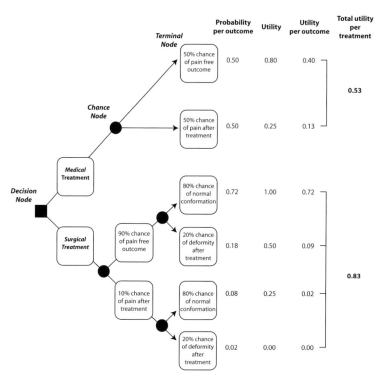

**Fig. 9.1**    A decision tree illustrating the analysis of a hypothetical decision to choose between a medical and a surgical treatment

A, B and C is £40, £30 and £20 respectively. There is a standard default cost, when further treatment is necessary, of £100 to achieve a recovery. The expected costs of the outcomes are computed from multiplying the probability of the outcome with the cost of the outcome. For example, with mastitis Tx A recovery is expected in 80% of cases and the cost of the treatment is £40 so that the expected cost is £32. To obtain the average cost of a specific intervention the expected outcomes for each intervention are summed. For example, with mastitis Tx A the expected cost of recovery is £32 and the expected cost for the initial cost plus the cost of further treatment is £28 (0.2 (£40 + £100)). The expected costs of the interventions can then be compared. In this case the expected costs of each intervention are Tx A (£60), Tx B (£70) and Tx C (£80), respectively. Mastitis Tx A is the best economic choice.

Figure 9.3 illustrates an economic decision analysis tree for three alternative treatments, with different costs and outcome probabilities, that may be used for a left displaced abomasum in a dairy cow. This analysis has been adapted from Feltrow (1985). In this condition recovery is not inevitable so that selecting the best option has to take into account the cost of slaughter and replacement, to produce a net value of the outcome. The outcome probabilities were sourced as

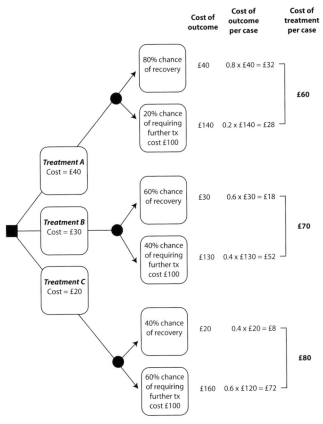

**Fig. 9.2** A decision tree illustrating the comparison of three hypothetical treatments for bovine mastitis incorporating a financial analysis of the outcomes

follows: rolling the cow (estimated by the authors), toggle method (Sterner and Grymer 1982), and omentoplexy (Saint Jean *et al.* 1987). The costings used were estimated by the authors. The decision tree yields total net values of £731, £745 and £756 for the rolling, omentoplexy and toggle methods, respectively, indicating that the toggle method is the method with the highest cost–benefit.

### 9.3.9  *Decision analysis tree of diagnostic tests*

Decision tree analysis is most commonly used to evaluate decisions at a herd or population level for disease eradication and control programmes (Smith and Slenning 2000).

Figure 9.4 illustrates how decision analysis can be used to deal with uncertainty in diagnostic testing. In this example, two tests are compared when used as a herd-screening test for infection with *Mycobacterium avium paratuberculosis*

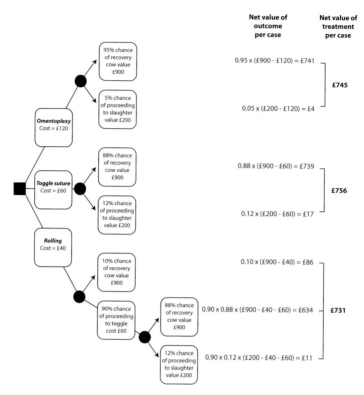

**Fig. 9.3**   A decision tree illustrating the analysis of different treatments for left displaced abomasum in dairy cows incorporating a financial analysis of the outcomes

(Johne's disease). The tests used in identification of subclinically infected animals have different probabilities for each outcome which makes comparisons and choices complex. The outcomes from a diagnostic test are the true positive animals, the false positive animals, the true negative animals and the false negative animals. By assigning a net value to each of these outcomes it is possible to derive a total net value for each method of testing in the presence of an assumed prevalence of disease in the herd. By doing so, the test with the greatest cost–benefit can be identified. The factors to consider, and the assumptions that have to be made to derive the net outcomes, are complex, and sometimes difficult to estimate accurately. In this case hypothetical estimates have been applied to demonstrate the methodology. It is instructive to consider some of the factors with regards to the four possible outcomes, as follows.

### False positives

Positive animals would be culled incurring a cost of replacement (minus the slaughter value) for no conceivable gain.

Herd size = 100
True prevalence = 0.02 (i.e. 2 cases in herd)

## Complement Fixation Test (CFT)

CFT sensitivity = 0.56
CFT specificity = 0.96

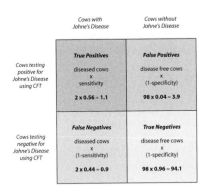

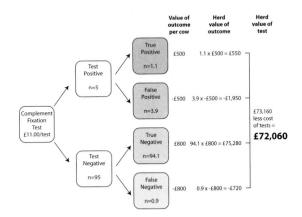

## ELISA Test for Antibodies

ELISA sensitivity = 0.60
ELISA specificity = 0.99

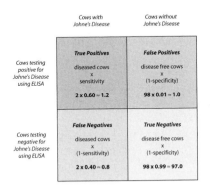

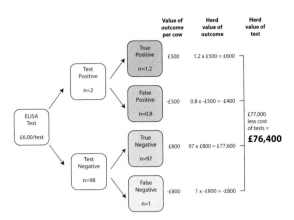

**Fig. 9.4** The calculation of the cost–benefit analyses of using two different tests for Johne's disease in a herd of cattle

## True positives

- These animals would also be culled, incurring the cost of replacement
- There would be a saving of losses avoided as a result of disease.

## False negatives

- Infected animals would be retained in herd
- There would be the cost of disease in a loss of production/carcass value
- Losses could also be attributed to the infection of new stock
- A further loss would be due to the infected status of the herd.

## True negatives

Value is added in this circumstance, as these animals are not infectious.

Decision trees can be used to investigate the impact of serial and parallel testing provided that values for conditional covariance are available.

In this scenario the ELISA test is the preferred option due to the higher herd value (£76 400).

### 9.3.10   Pay-off tables

Estimates or assumptions regarding the value of variables (e.g. prevalence) which influence the outcome may be made if their true value is uncertain. The outcome will therefore have more than one value assigned to it and a choice has to be made regarding the decision criterion to be used in the selection of which strategy, or test, to adopt.

#### MAXIMAX and MAXIMIN

Table 9.1 illustrates the cost–benefit of a whole-herd test for four tests at different disease prevalence levels. There are several established decision criteria that can be used. One approach is to identify the test which gives the highest financial return when the best financial returns from each test are compared. This is known as the MAXIMAX criterion and represents the most optimistic

**Table 9.1**   Cost–benefit of whole-herd testing of four tests at four different prevalences of disease.

|        | Prevalence | | | |
|--------|------|------|------|------|
| Test   | 0%   | 1%   | 5%   | 10%  |
| Test A | £3000 | £2000 | £1000 | £850 |
| Test B | £2500 | £2000 | £900 | £800 |
| Test C | £3100 | £2300 | £1100 | £1000 |
| Test D | £3500 | £2400 | £1300 | £900 |

outcome with regard to the financial return. A related approach is to identify the test that gives the highest financial return when the worst financial returns from each test are compared. This is known as the MAXIMIN criterion and represents the most pessimistic view with regard to the financial return. These two criteria are illustrated in table 9.2. Test D fulfils the MAXIMAX criterion and Test C fulfils the MAXIMIN criteria.

**Table 9.2**   Maximum and minimum cost–benefit for the four tests when four levels of prevalence, 0%, 1%, 5% and 10%, are considered.

| Test | Minimum | Maximum |
|------|---------|---------|
| Test A | £850 | £3000 |
| Test B | £800 | £2500 |
| Test C | **£1000 (MAXIMIN)** | £3100 |
| Test D | £900 | **£3500 (MAXIMAX)** |

## MINIMAX regret criterion

A third approach is called the MINIMAX regret decision criterion. This is illustrated in table 9.3. The money lost, compared to the best strategy, for each value of the variable is obtained for each test. For example, with 0% prevalence Test D is the best strategy, as the financial return is the highest. The opportunity cost is the difference between the value for Test D and the comparative test. The opportunity cost of using the other tests instead of Test D at 0% is shown in brackets. The highest opportunity cost for each test across all the different prevalences is identified. The test with the lowest 'maximum regret' cost is the strategy chosen, in this case Test D. This means that compared to the best possible strategy, whatever the prevalence, the maximum difference in the value of the outcome would be £100.

## Likelihood or expected money value criterion

If we wished to add another layer of sophistication to the decision-making process we could consider the likelihood of the different prevalences. It may be

**Table 9.3**   MINIMAX regret decision for Tests A, B, C and D at the levels of prevalence 0%, 1%, 5% and 10%.

| Test | Prevalence | | | | Max regret |
|------|------|------|------|------|------------|
| | 0% | 1% | 5% | 10% | |
| Test A | £3000 (£500) | £2000 (£400) | £1000 (£300) | £850 (£300) | £500 |
| Test B | £2500 (£1000) | £2000 (£400) | £900 (£400) | £800 (£200) | £1000 |
| Test C | £3100 (£400) | £2300 (£100) | £1100 (£200) | £1000 (best) | £400 |
| Test D | £3500 (best) | £2400 (best) | £1300 (best) | £900 (£100) | **£100** |

possible to estimate the probability of each value of the variable occurring (prevalence in this example). Let us assume that the probability of the prevalences are: 0% prevalence = 0.3, 1% prevalence = 0.4, 5% prevalence = 0.2, and 10% prevalence = 0.1. The value for each cell within each prevalence category is given by the value of the cell given in table 9.1 multiplied by the probability of that prevalence occurring. This value is termed the expected money value (EMV). This is shown in table 9.4.

**Table 9.4**   Expected money values of the Tests A, B, C and D with prevalences and probabilities of those prevalences of 0% (0.3), 1% (0.4), 5% (0.2) and 10% (0.1).

| Test | Prevalence (probability) | | | |
|---|---|---|---|---|
| | 0% (0.3) | 1% (0.4) | 5% (0.2) | 10% (0.1) |
| Test A | £3000 × 0.3 = £900 | £2000 × 0.4 = £800 | £1000 × 0.2 = £200 | £850 × 0.1 = £85 |
| Test B | £2500 × 0.3 = £750 | £2000 × 0.4 = £800 | £900 × 0.2 = £180 | £800 × 0.1 = £80 |
| Test C | £3100 × 0.3 = £930 | £2300 × 0.4 = £920 | £1100 × 0.2 = £220 | £1000 × 0.1 = £100 |
| Test D | £3500 × 0.3 = £1050 | £2400 × 0.4 = £960 | £1300 × 0.2 = £260 | £900 × 0.1 = £90 |

Applying the MAXIMIN criterion and MAXIMAX criterion to the EMVs described in table 9.5 Test C is the MAXIMIN Test and Test D is the MAXIMAX Test. The MINIMAX regret criterion can also be applied to the EMV. This is shown in table 9.6.

**Table 9.5**   Maximum and minimum cost benefit for Tests A, B, C and D when four levels of prevalence, 0%, 1%, 5% and 10%, are considered using expected monetary value criterion.

| Test | Minimum | Maximum |
|---|---|---|
| Test A | £85 | £900 |
| Test B | £80 | £800 |
| Test C | **£100 MAXIMIN** | £930 |
| Test D | £90 | **£1050 MAXIMAX** |

The test with the lowest maximum regret cost is the strategy chosen, in this case Test D. This means that compared to the best possible strategy whatever the prevalence the maximum difference in the value of the outcome would be £40.

Sensitivity analysis can be used to monitor the impact of changes of the value of selected variables where uncertainty exists.

**Table 9.6** EMV regret criterion.

| Test | 0% (0.3) | 1% (0.4) | 5% (0.2) | 10% (0.1) | Maximum EMV regret |
|------|----------|----------|----------|-----------|--------------------|
| Test A | £900 (£150) | £800 (£160) | £200 (£60) | £85 (£15) | £160 |
| Test B | £750 (£300) | £800 (£160) | £180 (£80) | £80 (£20) | £300 |
| Test C | £930 (£120) | £920 (£40) | £220 (£40) | £100 (£0) | £120 |
| Test D | £1050 (£0) | £960 (£0) | £260 (£0) | £90 (£10) | **£40 MINIMAX** |

### 9.3.11 User checklist for clinical decision analysis

*Are the results valid?*

- Were all the important strategies and outcomes included?
- Was an explicit and sensible process used to identify, select and combine the evidence into probabilities?
- Were the utilities obtained in an explicit and sensible way from credible sources?
- Was the potential impact of any uncertainty in the evidence determined?

*What are the results?*

- Does one strategy result in a clinically/economically important gain?
- How strong is the evidence used in the analysis?
- Could the uncertainty in the evidence change the result?

*Are the results applicable to my scenario?*

- Do the probability estimates apply to my patient/situation?
- Do the utilities reflect how my owner would value the outcomes of the decision?

## 9.4 Testing and treating thresholds

Decision analysis can be used to decide if a patient should undergo a diagnostic test and/or treatment.

In this analysis, the probability of disease in a patient (the pre-test probability, derived from the prevalence), is compared with the testing threshold value and the treatment threshold value.

Values for the following five factors are required to compute the testing and treatment thresholds:

- Benefit of therapy
- Risk or cost of therapy
- Risk of the test

- Sensitivity of the test
- Specificity of the test.

The values of the benefit, risk of therapy and risk of test can either be in terms of:

- cost (£)
- the likelihood of a favourable outcome (0–1.0).

Testing threshold =

$$\frac{((1 - \text{specificity}) \times \text{risk of therapy}) + \text{risk of test}}{((1 - \text{specificity}) \times \text{risk of therapy}) + (\text{sensitivity} \times \text{benefit of therapy})}$$

Treatment threshold =

$$\frac{(\text{specificity} \times \text{risk of therapy}) - \text{risk of test}}{(\text{specificity} \times \text{risk of therapy}) + ((1 - \text{sensitivity}) \times \text{benefit of therapy})}$$

The values obtained whether using costs or likelihoods are in the range 0–1.0. The values for the testing and treating thresholds are then compared with the probability of disease in a patient (the pre-test probability) expressed as a likelihood (range 0–1.0). There are three possible outcomes:

(1) Probability of disease in the patient is below the testing threshold. With this result both the treatment and the test should be withheld. The risk or cost of the test outweighs the benefit of the test diagnostic information.
(2) Probability of disease in the patient is between the testing and treating threshold (the testing band). The test should be performed, and treatment guided by the test result.
(3) Probability of disease in the patient is above the treating threshold. Treatment should be given without testing, as the diagnostic test result will not change the action.

These outcomes are illustrated in figure 9.5.

## 9.4.1   *General properties of testing and treating thresholds*

- Testing and treating thresholds decrease as the risk of therapy decreases or as the benefit of therapy increases

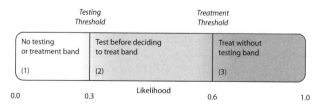

**Fig. 9.5**   A diagrammatic representation of thresholds, and testing and treatment bands

- Testing and treating thresholds both increase as the risk of therapy increases or as the benefit of therapy decreases
- The testing band widens as the risk of testing decreases or as the sensitivity and specificity increase
- The testing band narrows as the risk of testing increases or as the sensitivity and specificity decrease.

Worked veterinary examples are provided by Smith (1991). Treatment and testing thresholds are covered in considerable detail by Friedland *et al.* (1998).

In human medicine, decision analysis has been used to provide evidence-based guidelines for patients in a defined category. These guidelines provide management strategies that deliver the highest expected utility and the lowest unfavourable outcome to patients. While there is insufficient reliable data to enable the production of useful guidelines across a broad range of conditions, this approach could be applied to some clinical situations in veterinary medicine, and at the very least form a basis for discussion of their potential value.

In more general terms, the utility attached to each outcome may be economic or may be owner derived. Whichever is used, a best choice can be identified. The variables within the decision tree can be changed to monitor the impact on the total net value of the outcomes. Spreadsheets (e.g. Microsoft® Excel) can be used to advantage so that a wide range of inputs can be tested to discover the impact on the outputs.

For a more detailed discussion on veterinary decision analysis see Collins and Morgan (1991), Smith (1993), Smith and Slenning (2000) and Radostits *et al.* (2000).

## 9.5 Modelling

Many of the methods for decision analysis described above are a simple form of mathematical modelling. Mathematical models try to recreate a real-world situation using a series of mathematical relationships. Most of us use a mathematical model to set our budgets for the year. The input variables are our projected income and expenditure which we estimate from our previous year's experience, and we ask questions of the model such as whether or not we can afford to hire a new assistant, or buy a new endoscope.

There has been increasing use of modelling within veterinary medicine to look at infectious diseases and their control. These dynamic models which encompass changes over time are used to predict events and to assess the relative merits of alternative control strategies. In doing so, they can provide evidence for decision making. The complete model can be very complex, but it can be broken down into a number (possibly very large) of simple mathematical relationships and initial parameter values.

The choice of which parameters to include is an important one. There are usually numerous potential parameters that may influence the outcome. Parameters that do, and do not, contribute to the problem solving can be identified by a sensitivity analysis, in which the value of a parameter is varied while the others are kept constant. Changes to the outcome are monitored. If there is no significant change in the outcome then the parameter may be removed from the model. If there is a large change in the outcome then the parameter is likely to be retained.

Most models for applied veterinary practice produce a quantitative outcome. There are two main types of quantitative model: deterministic and non-deterministic. Deterministic models use a single set of values for the parameters, and these give a single outcome value. Non-deterministic models use a set of conditions which takes into account the probability of each parameter value. Calculations are made for all the values of each parameter and the results collated, taking into account the different weighting of each result. The number of runs required for all the parameter values generated by probabilistic models can be very large, and powerful computers are required to reduce the time needed to complete the computations.

Models can be broadly divided into mechanistic or empirical models. Mechanistic models are based upon known and hypothesised biological relationships, whereas empirical models are based upon observed relationships, with no attempt to explain the underlying association.

The quality of the model depends upon how closely it simulates the real world. This requires a process of model validation. Testing to measure the accuracy of the model over a range of starting circumstances is a crucial step in providing evidence for the usefulness of the model. The more complex the situation that we are trying to model, the less likely it is to match the real world. If it were easy, we would be able to use such models to predict the winners of horse races, and retire on our winnings! On the other hand, our best attempts at mathematical modelling may be our only way of estimating the future patterns of epidemics of diseases. Models are being used to predict the most important factors in the spread of foot and mouth disease, and their use was influential in the outbreak in the UK in 2001. At a smaller scale, epidemiological models have been used to indicate critical control points in the management of *Staphylococcus aureus* infection in a herd.

The majority of models are coded using basic programming languages such as Fortran or C++, using structured programming language such as Matlab or specifically developed packages such as Model Maker.

### 9.5.1   *Modelling herd infection dynamics* (Skukken *et al.* 2002)

The dynamics of infectious diseases can be represented by state transition models. The animals in the herd fall into one of three states: susceptible to infection, infectious or resistant. BHV1 is an example. Susceptible animals would be sero-negative, infectious animals would be shedding virus, and resistant animals are sero-positive.

The transitions between states can be represented as:

Change of susceptibles with time $\dfrac{dS}{dt} = +\mu N - \beta SI - \mu S$

Change of infected with time $\dfrac{dI}{dt} = +\beta SI - \alpha I - \mu I$

Change of resistant with time $\dfrac{dR}{dt} = \alpha I - \mu R$

where S = susceptible; I = infectious; R = resistant;
$\mu$ = the rate of birth or death (assuming constant population size N);
$\beta$ = the rate of contact between S and I animals multiplied by the probability that the contact leads to infection;
$\alpha$ = the rate of moving from infectious to resistant.

An outbreak of BHV1 had the values:

$\mu = 0.033$
$\beta = 0.0043$
$\alpha = 0.067.$

The progress of an outbreak can be presented graphically (figure 9.6).

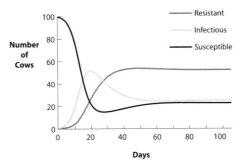

**Fig. 9.6** A graph showing the results of running a deterministic state transition model for BHV1 in a herd of cows. The number of susceptible, infectious, and resistant animals are shown against time

This graph shows the number of animals over time in the three categories Susceptible, Infectious and Resistant. The Reproduction Ratio (R) is a key parameter in understanding the herd dynamics. The critical value for R is 1 indicating that an infection leads to one new infection, thus maintaining endemic stability. When R is greater than 1 an exponential growth of infected individuals occurs, while a value of less than 1 leads to eventual extinction of the infection.

$$R = \left(\frac{\beta}{\mu + \alpha}\right) \times \frac{S}{NR_0}$$

at the start of the outbreak

$$R = R_0 \times \frac{S}{N}$$

$$R = R_0$$

$R_0$ is the number of new infections resulting from a single infected individual in a fully susceptible population.

### 9.5.2   *Modelling and the control of foot and mouth disease*

Three models were used to inform policy in the foot and mouth disease (FMD) outbreak. They were the Imperial College model (deterministic), the Cambridge/Edinburgh combined model (non-deterministic) and the VLA model (non-deterministic). The Imperial College model used infectiousness, susceptibility and transmissibility. The Cambridge/Edinburgh models used three parameters (infectiousness, susceptibility and transmissibility) with 100 simulation runs daily in contrast to the VLA model which used over 50 parameters, with five simulation runs daily. The models were used to investigate two control strategies culling and vaccination.

The culling control strategy investigated the area of cull, and the speed of cull in relation to the control of infection. In the Imperial College model the progress of the disease was estimated from the value of $R_0$. $R_0$ is the transmission potential of the infectious agent and measures the average number of secondarily infected farms derived from a primary source of infection in a susceptible group of farms. If $R_0$ is <1 then there will be no further spread of disease and the disease is assumed to be under control. It is estimated, using the contact data, by multiplying the average number of infectious days by the average number of farms infected, per infectious day. The Imperial College model showed that $R_0$ was sensitive to delays in identifying, reporting and confirming the presence of disease, and the speed by which the infected farm could be culled. $R_0$ could be reduced if the animals on an infected premises could be slaughtered within 24 hours without waiting for laboratory confirmation but that it would still remain >1. To reduce $R_0$ <1 contiguous premises had to be culled within 48 hours of the infected premise cull.

The Cambridge/Edinburgh model showed similar results in that the speed of identification and culling were important. This model also predicted the long tail-off of this epidemic. The VLA model showed that pre-emptive slaughtering of an average of 1.4 farms for every infected farm would result in eradication of the disease by the end of October 2001 at the latest which was in accordance with the other models.

As a result of these models, control strategies were implemented to facilitate the rapid slaughtering of infected and contiguous premises.

### 9.5.3 *Modelling* Staphylococcus aureus *infection in a herd*

This is a deterministic state transition model (Zadocks 2002) summarised in figure 9.7. It is mechanistic. Parameter estimates for the transition rates between states (e.g. the cure rate for clinical cases, remission rates from clinical to subclinical states) are used to predict prevalence of infected quarters over time. The outcome when using different control strategies can be generated by changing the values of the parameters. Thus a range of strategies can be tested and the most appropriate control strategy chosen for the control and eradication of *Staphylococcus aureus*.

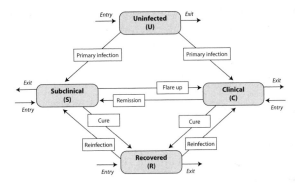

**Fig. 9.7** A diagrammatic representation of a deterministic state transition model for *Staphylococcus aureus* infection in a herd of dairy cows

### 9.5.4 *User guide to models*

- What are the assumptions used in the model and are these biologically plausible?
- What type of model is being described – deterministic or non-deterministic?
- What are the estimates of the parameter values based upon?
- How was the model validated?
- Is the output important in my decision making?
- Does the model represent my 'real world'?
- Is the model output strategic in a general qualitative sense (e.g. cull contiguous herds of an FMD infected herd within 24 hours) or does it have specific, tangible, quantifiable results (e.g. replacing scrapie susceptible rams with scrapie resistant rams will produce a resistant flock in X years)?

## 9.6 Economic analysis

This is an important and complex subject in farm animal practice. The direct and indirect cost of disease, suboptimal fertility and production are important factors in decision analysis and intervention. Performance indicators for comparative purposes are vital for identifying and characterising problems and devising corrective strategies.

Farmers are eager to obtain information regarding their potential to increase profit margins (or reduce losses) and require evidence-based assessments of the cost–benefit of expensive intervention strategies. Marketing of herd health plans and farm animal veterinary practice can only be achieved if there is good evidence to support the costs and benefits proposed. Recording schemes combined with detailed economic analysis can provide accurate values to assess the cost of disease or suboptimal production and the cost–benefit of interventions. Economic evaluation can therefore be made based upon the best available evidence that the values used are valid at the farm level.

Economic studies and analyses of dairy cow fertility, health and productivity from a large number of UK herds have been published (Esslemont and Kossaibati 2000, 2002). They provide economic analyses of a range of conditions. The surveys analyse the comparative financial performances of different percentiles of the recorded herds. They also report the incidence of key diseases, and the values of key fertility indices, for the different percentiles. For example, the best 10% of herds and the bottom 10% of herds can be compared.

The direct costs associated with 30 different endemic diseases of farm animals in Great Britain have been estimated (13 cattle, 5 swine, 7 sheep and 5 poultry) (Bennett *et al.* 1999). Simple spreadsheet models of each disease were constructed. The value of key disease parameters were estimated from published literature, the Veterinary Investigation Diagnosis Analysis System, and unpublished research from the Veterinary Laboratories Agency. Each spreadsheet had explanatory notes indicating the derivations of the parameter values and the calculations used. The spreadsheet models, accompanying notes and disease reports (literature review) are available in full on the Internet at the website address: www.rdg.ac.uk/livestockdisea/

### 9.6.1 Partial budgets and cost–benefit analysis

The cost of decisions regarding control or treatment strategies is often the most important factor in deciding upon implementation in farm animals. It is not a simple task to quantify the losses from diseases. Quantification of the economic losses from disease is usually performed by simple partial budgeting, or using cost–benefit analysis techniques.

## Partial budgeting

This involves identifying those returns and costs that will change as a result of a specific intervention. These may include:

(1)  additional returns
(2)  reduced costs
(3)  returns forgone
(4)  extra costs.

The net return = (1 + 2) − (3 + 4)

## Cost–benefit analysis

This is a method of producing a cost–benefit ratio. In the simplest cost–benefit analysis the financial benefits (B) are divided by the costs (C). The ratio of the benefits to the costs (B/C) is the cost–benefit ratio. In general the cost–benefit of veterinary services to the farmer is between 200% and 500%, although with herd health programmes this can be much higher.

Because benefits and costs do not occur simultaneously they cannot be compared directly without adjusting for the time value of money.

The formula used to calculate the present value (PV) of a future cost or benefit (FV) where r is the annual rate of interest (%) and n is the number of years in the future is:

$$PV = \frac{FV}{\left(1 + \frac{r}{100}\right)^n}$$

The interest rate used in the cost–benefit analysis is called the discount rate, since it makes future values smaller than present values as this money will earn no interest over time. The higher the discount rate, or the longer the time to accrue benefit, the smaller the present value. The discount rate (e.g. 5%) usually used is called the real interest rate, and is the difference between the market rate of interest (e.g. 9%) and the inflation rate (e.g. 4%).

Once the expected flow of costs and benefits have been calculated allowing for the time at which they occur, three decision criteria may then be used to make a decision.

(1)  Net present value (benefits)

Total present value − total present costs

This represents the value of benefits of the strategy at current prices.

(2)  Benefit–cost ratio (B/C ratio)

Total present value of benefits/total present value of costs

This represents the relative size of the costs and benefits but gives no indication of the scale of investment required.

(3)   Internal rate of return (IRR)

This is the interest rate that would make the total present value of the benefits equal to that of the costs over the designated time period. This avoids having the use of a discount rate. The IRR cannot be defined by formula but is obtained by trial and error.

### 9.6.2   *User guide to economic analysis*

- Are the direct and indirect costs of any intervention included in the costings used?
- What are the sources of the values used?
- Are the values used still current?
- Has the present value been adjusted for the time value of money if the benefits occur over time?

## 9.7   Medline search functions

When searching for relevant papers on Pubmed the following Medline terms should be of use:

- Decision support techniques [MH]
- Cost–benefit analysis [MH]
- Decision analysis [ti].

## References and further reading

Bennett, R.M., Christiansen, K. and Clifton-Hadley, R.S. (1999) Direct costs of endemic diseases of farm animals in Great Britain. *Veterinary Record* **145**, 376–7.

Collins, M.T. and Morgan, I.R. (1991) Economic decision analysis model of a paratuberculosis test and cull program. *Journal of the American Veterinary Medical Association* **199** (12), 1724–9.

Esslemont, R.J. and Kossaibati, M.A. (2000) Dairy farming systems: husbandry, economics and recording. In *The Health of Dairy Cattle* (ed. Andrews, A.H.). Blackwell Science, Oxford.

Esslemont, R.J. and Kossaibati, M.A. (2002) The costs of poor fertility and disease. In *UK Dairy Herds*, Intervet, Milton Keynes.

Feltrow, J. (1985) Economic decisions in veterinary practice: a method for field use. *Journal of the American Veterinary Medical Association* **186** (8), 792–7.

Friedland, D.J, Go, A.S., Davoran, J.B. *et al.* (1998) *Evidence-based Medicine: A framework for clinical practice.* Lange Medical Books/McGraw-Hill, New York.

Haywood, S. and Haywood, G. (2002) Modelling and FMD. *BCVA Congress Times* 16–18 July, 2002.

Radostits, O.M., Gay, C.G., Blood, D.C., Hinchcliff, K.W. (2000) Clinical examination and making a diagnosis. In *Veterinary Medicine*, Radostits, O.M. (ed.). Saunders, London, p. 31.

Ridge, S.E., Morgan, I.R., Sockett, D.C. *et al.* (1991) Comparison of Johne's absorbed EIA and complement-fixation test for the diagnosis of Johne's disease in cattle. *Australian Veterinary Journal* **68** (8), 253–7.

Saint Jean, C.D., Hull, B.L., Hoffsis, G.F. and Rings, M.D. (1987) Comparison of different surgical techniques for the correction of abomasal problems. *Compendium Continuing Education Food Animal* **9** (11), F377–82.

Skukken, Y.H., van Schaik, G. and Zadoks, R.N. (2002) Handling of infectious herd problems: role of the individual in herd and population. In *Recent Developments and Perspectives in Bovine Medicine*, XXII World Buiatrics Congress 2002. Klinik für Rinderkrankheiten, Tierärztliche Hochschule, Hannover.

Smith, R.D. (1995) *Veterinary Clinical Epidemiology*. Butterworth-Heinemann, London.

Smith, R.D. (1993) Decision analysis in the evaluation of diagnostic tests. *Journal of the American Veterinary Medical Association* **203** (8), 1184–92.

Smith, R.D. and Slenning, B.D. (2000) Decision analysis: dealing with uncertainty in diagnostic testing. *Preventive Veterinary Medicine* **45** (1–2), 139–62.

Sterner, K.E. and Grymer, J. (1982) Closed suture techniques using the bar-suture for correction of left displaced abomasum – a review of 100 cases. *Bovine Practitioner* **17**, 80–84.

Zadocks, R.N. (2002) Molecular and mathematical epidemiology of *Staphylococcus aureus* and *Streptococcus uberis* in dairy herds. PhD thesis, Utrecht University, The Netherlands.

## Review questions

Answers on page 205

**1** *Decision trees are composed of:*

    (a)   Decision nodes
    (b)   Chance nodes
    (c)   Terminal nodes
    (d)   All of these.

**2** *Decision tree decision nodes are nodes where:*

    (a)   A conscious decision between two or more options is made
    (b)   No decisions are made; likelihoods are attached to each outcome derived from the chance node. The likelihoods or probabilities of the outcomes emanating from a chance node add up to 1.0 or 100% respectively
    (c)   Utilities are attached to these nodes to indicate the value attached to the outcome by the owner.

**3** *Decision tree chance nodes are nodes where:*

    (a)   A conscious decision between two or more options is made
    (b)   No decisions are made; likelihoods are attached to each outcome derived from the chance node. The likelihoods or probabilities of the outcomes emanating from a chance node add up to 1.0 or 100%, respectively
    (c)   Utilities are attached to these nodes to indicate the value attached to the outcome by the owner.

**4** *Decision tree terminal nodes are nodes where:*

    (a)   A conscious decision between two or more options is made
    (b)   No decisions are made; likelihoods are attached to each outcome derived from the chance node. The likelihoods or probabilities of the outcomes emanating from a chance node add up to 1.0 or 100%, respectively
    (c)   Utilities are attached to these nodes to indicate the value attached to the outcome by the owner.

**5** *Owner utilities can be obtained by using:*

    (a)   Dialogue
    (b)   Visual analogue scales
    (c)   Time trade-off calculations
    (d)   Standard gamble techniques
    (e)   All of the above.

**6** *When calculating treatment and testing thresholds possible outcomes may be:*

(a) Probability of disease in the patient is below the testing threshold
(b) Probability of disease in the patient is between the testing and treating threshold (the testing band)
(c) Probability of disease in the patient is above the treating threshold
(d) (a) or (b) or (c).

**7** *Sensitivity analysis in modelling is:*

(a) The evaluation of the impact of changing the value of a variable, or variables, on the model results
(b) The number of times the model was correct
(c) A measure of how good the model is.

**8** *In cost–benefit analysis total present value – total present costs is called the:*

(a) Net present value (benefits)
(b) Benefit–cost ratio (B/C ratio)
(c) Internal rate of return (IRR).

**9** *In cost–benefit analysis, total present value of benefits/total present value of costs ratio is called:*

(a) Net present value (benefits)
(b) Benefit–cost ratio (B/C ratio)
(c) Internal rate of return (IRR).

**10** *There are several established decision criteria that can be used. One approach is to identify the test which gives the highest financial return when the best financial returns from each test are compared. This is called:*

(a) MAXIMAX
(b) MAXIMIN.

# 10

# EBVM: EDUCATION AND FUTURE NEEDS

It is instructive to describe the current state of EBM as this provides useful guidelines for the development of EBVM particularly regarding the accessibility to evidence from the literature.

## 10.1 EBM in medical education

Walk into any medical bookshop and you will see shelves full of evidence-based books in every discipline represented. Look on the Internet and you will find post-graduate courses available several times a year to meet the demand. Numerous books cover the topic of EBM and some have become even more specialised by dealing only with how to critically appraise the literature. Undergraduate curricula are now including EBM, with ever increasing priority being given to it.

## 10.2 Resources for the practice of EBM

Outlined below are some of the developments that have enabled EBM to become a reality in everyday medical practice.

### 10.2.1 Critically appraised topics (CATs)

There are now a number of Internet sites that contain a database of CATs.

A CAT is a short summary of the evidence to a focused clinical question. The preparation of a CAT enables this information to be shared or used at a later date. CATs are a summary of one paper, they can be wrong and they quickly become redundant as new evidence becomes available. Standard protocols have been produced regarding the format of CATs. Any qualified practitioners may submit CATs to dedicated websites such as that hosted by the Centre for Evidence-based Medicine at Oxford (minerva.minervation.com/cebm/docs/catbank.html). This is illustrated in figure 10.1. Some EBM centres use the acronym POEM (Patient Orientated Evidence that Matters) as an alternative to CAT.

### 10.2.2 High quality systematic reviews

Systematic reviews of the literature designed to answer a specific clinical question represent a form of secondary scientific literature with a very high evidence value. They enable evidence to be located quickly, in a summarised form, with an objective science-based opinion addressing the quality of the evidence presented. In human medicine, dedicated resources exist to fulfil this

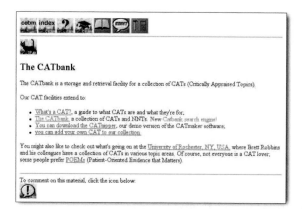

**Fig. 10.1**   The CATbank page from the website of the Centre for Evidence-based Medicine at Oxford

need. The Cochrane Library is a good example of a database of systematic reviews.

### 10.2.3   The Cochrane Library (www.cochrane.de)

The Cochrane Library contains over 1000 systematic reviews (figure 10.2). A good systematic review will summarise all the high quality published, and sometimes unpublished, research around a specific clinical question. It is an international collaboration. The reviews consider all types of methodology and use explicit criteria for the inclusion and analysis of trials in the review. The evidence for clinical recommendations is summarised. The reviews are avail-

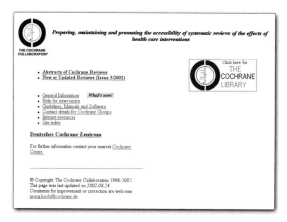

**Fig. 10.2**   The front page of the Cochrane Collaboration website

able in an easy to search format on the Internet and CD-ROM, as well as hard copy. The reviews are frequently updated to remain current.

### 10.2.4 *Secondary journals (e.g. EBM)*

Secondary journals to support the practice of EBM have developed in human medicine. Secondary journals publish structured abstracts summarising the best quality evidence and most clinically useful recent research from the literature.

## 10.3 EBM in veterinary education

### 10.3.1 *Evidence-based veterinary toolkit*

It is now time to accept that there is a range of skills that are required to provide the best practice for our patients that many of us have not yet acquired. These skills include computer skills, an understanding of experimental design, the ability to transform clinical questions into questions to which the answer may be found in the literature, and an ability to understand and critically appraise the evidence being presented. We need to have an evidence-based veterinary medicine toolkit in our armoury of professional skills. There is an urgent need to develop a suitable EBVM syllabus for undergraduates, and to provide appropriate CPD courses for post-graduates.

### 10.3.2 *Finding out what is in the literature and what is not in the literature*

One argument that can be used against the practice of EBVM is that there is insufficient depth and breadth in the veterinary scientific literature. However, there is no excuse for failing to search for the best evidence. When we search for evidence but fail to find it, we identify deficits that prevent us from making the best decisions. If, as practitioners, we share our experiences of searching the literature, apart from sharing the work (possibly using CATs), a broad practitioner base can provide a powerful voice to direct the scientific effort to where it is required.

## 10.4 What resources do we need for the practice of EBVM?

We also need competently produced systematic reviews of the past and present literature using an explicit methodology made available on the Internet. As we are a small profession, the greater the collaboration on a worldwide basis, the greater will be the resources.

It is clear that if EBVM is to succeed we need:

- Systematic reviews
- Secondary journals
- A central database of CATs
- More clinical trials
- Education at all levels in EBVM skills
- Audit of commonly asked questions for which there is poor evidence to identify priority areas for clinical research and systematic review.

## 10.5    Clinical (EBVM) audits in veterinary practice

### 10.5.1    What is a clinical audit?

Clinical audit has been defined as:

'The systematic critical analysis of the quality of medical care, including the procedures used for diagnosis and treatment, the use of resources and the resulting outcome and quality of life for the patient.' (DoH 1998)

The need to make clinical audits evidence-based has been stated:

'Clinical audit must always be evidence-based to ensure that clinical practice and decisions to change it are based upon the best possible evidence of effectiveness.' (DoH 1998)

### 10.5.2    Why do we need a clinical audit?

It is important to be able to assure clients and peers that the expertise and service offered is safe, effective and efficient. Clinical audit is a process used by health professionals to assess, evaluate and improve patient care. The process identifies deficiencies and monitors the outcome of any changes made to address these deficiencies.

### 10.5.3    What has a clinical audit got to do with EBVM?

Clinical audits can be used to compare current practice with the best available evidence. It provides a methodology to assess if the best evidence-base medicine is being applied within the practice.

### 10.5.4    How do we carry out an EBVM audit?

Starting with a perceived important and common problem within the practice is useful to stimulate interest and motivate participants. Examples of possible topics in small animals may include: pyoderma, diabetes mellitus and congestive heart failure in dogs; chronic renal failure, miliary eczema and hyperthyroidism in cats. Examples in large animals may include laminitis, heaves (COPD) and melanomas in horses; toxic mastitis, endometritis and solar ulceration in cattle. The treatments and the outcomes derived from practice records should be compared with those available from the best evidence according to the published literature.

The criteria and selection of data must be systematic and it usually involves collation of data from computerised records. The method of retrieval must be simple and foolproof. Analysis may present trends or just provide information for comparison. Statistical analysis may be appropriate but is not essential.

### 10.5.5   Clinical audits and the future

In addition to professional revalidation and CPD requirements, clinical audits could provide a means for the profession (practices) to demonstrate to clients and peers that the expertise and service offered is safe, effective and efficient. In the latest edition of the *Manual of Standards for Small Animal Hospitals* produced by the British Veterinary Hospitals Association, there is a stipulation that veterinary hospitals must have a means of measuring clinical outcome, especially for common problems.

## 10.6   Other future developments

Below are some of the other likely future developments that are common to both EBM and EBVM.

It is likely that laboratory-based randomised controlled trials will become more difficult to perform due to concerns regarding the use of animals in experimentation.

Certain types of study such as case–control studies are likely to become easier to perform as a result of the use of computer-based records. Increased clinical data recording is likely to lead to a more quantitative approach to clinical signs, and likelihood ratios will be available for the clinical profiles of patients. Research is likely to become more patient/owner orientated as EBVM provides a stronger link between scientists and practitioners. It is likely that journals will no longer rely on the amateurish goodwill and inherent bias of peer reviewers, and professional full-time reviewers will be employed to critically appraise submitted papers.

The culture of acquiring knowledge and memorising facts is likely to change to a culture encouraging the retention of core facts and the rapid search for case-specific information. *Just in time knowledge acquisition* rather than *just in case knowledge memorising.* To this end, veterinary students will have to be taught the skills required to do this.

In order to achieve this, Valori (2001) states that there will be a need for:

- Fewer or more uniform databases
- Better indexing and tagging of controlled trials
- Tagging of discredited evidence
- Links to full text papers and reviews
- Voice-activated searches supported by artificial intelligence
- Uniformity in the format and criteria used to present summary and primary evidence
- Locally adapted guidelines (practice) from centrally tested evidence (universities, institutes and referral practices).

## References and further reading

Baden, D. and Heneghan, C. (2002) *Evidence-based Medicine Toolkit.* BMJ Books, London.

DoH (Department of Health) (1998) *A First Class Service.* HMSO, London.

Mosedale, P. (1998) Introducing clinical audit to veterinary practice. *In Practice* **20** (1), 40–2.

Rayment, K. (2002) Clinical audit – a means of evaluating quality. *In Practice* **24** (8), 481–4.

Valori, R.M. (2001) The future of EBM. In *Key Topics in Evidence-based Medicine* (ed. McGovern, D.P.B., Valori, R.M., Summerskill, W.S.M. and Levi, M.). Bios Scientific Publications Ltd, Oxford.

# GLOSSARY

# BIBLIOGRAPHY

# ANSWERS TO SELF-ASSESSMENT QUESTIONS

# INDEX

# GLOSSARY OF TERMS USED IN EBVM

**Absolute benefit increase (ABI)**: The absolute arithmetic difference in event rates when describing a positive outcome.

**Absolute risk increase (ARI)**: When the test treatment harms more animals than the control treatment (see Absolute risk reduction below).

**Absolute risk reduction (ARR)**: The difference in the event rate between untreated control animals (the CER, control event rate), and the treated animals (the EER, experimental event rate).

**Allocation concealed**: See Blinded and Blinding

**Association**: A link between two or more events, characteristics, or other variables for which there is statistical evidence. An association may be detected because of a direct causal link, an indirect causal link, or may have no causal link.

**Attributable risk**: Additional risk of disease is the exposed group over that in the unexposed group. If mammary cancer occurs in 1 of 3000 speyed bitches (fictitious numbers) and in 21 of 3000 intact bitches, the attributable risk leaving bitches entire is 20 in 3000.

**Bayes' theorem**: Describes the mathematical formula for updating the probability of some event as new evidence becomes available.

**Bayesian belief networks**: Use a mathematical technique to assess quantitatively the effect that different pieces of information will have on our belief in a variety of different outcomes. They take a number of pieces of evidence and consistently evaluate their joint significance to determine the relative plausibility of different hypotheses. It does this using a set of Bayes's rules (a mathematical rule to relate conditional probabilities) acting on a network of relationship between different observations and hypotheses. The numbers which a Bayesian network generates are known as beliefs because they describe the belief which we might have in different hypotheses given the observation of particular pieces of evidence.

**Bias**: Any factor in the design or execution of a trial, other than the intended intervention, which might affect the interpretation of the results.

**Blinded and Blinding**: A technique used in clinical trials to prevent bias arising from the participants' knowledge of the intervention. In a study described as blinded, the authors were deemed to have taken adequate measures to conceal allocation to study groups from those responsible for assessing animals for entry in the trial (e.g. formal randomisation; sequentially numbered, opaque, sealed envelopes; sealed envelopes from a closed bag; numbered or coded bottles or containers; drugs prepared by the pharmacy; or other descriptions that contain elements convincing of concealment).

**Blinded study** (may also be called a masked study): In single-blinded studies the animal/owner is unaware of which intervention is used. In double-blinded studies neither the observers nor the animal/owners know which intervention is used. In triple-blinded studies the statistical analysis of the results is also carried out without revealing which intervention was used (e.g. the statistician knows that animals received either treatment A or treatment B, but not what they were).

**Boolean search**: A means of combining search statements or sets using the logical operators 'OR' to expand a search and 'AND' to restrict a search to articles that contain two or more specified elements together used in searching databases or the Internet.

**Case–control study**: A study in which animals representing cases of a disease are compared with a matched group of animals without this disease in order to see if they were exposed to the putative cause (and the disease-free animals weren't). This type of study is normally retrospective.

**Case report or Case study**: The report of a single case. Although anecdotal case reports represent the first step in observational epidemiology (when a new disease occurs someone has to point it out). However, the requirement in post-graduate education for candidates to produce papers means that a lot of such papers are of little use or relevance to general veterinary practitioners.

**Case series**: A publication, normally a paper in a journal, in which a series of animals with an outcome of interest are described. No control groups are used in the analysis of any data presented. They represent a poor source of evidence in scientific terms.

**Central tendency**: The middle of a distribution. Described by mean, median and mode.

**Chance**: Random variation. Difference between the outcomes from a sample of the population and the true value obtained from looking at the outcomes from the entire population. Statistical methods are used to estimate the probability that chance alone accounts for the differences in outcomes.

**Clinical significance** (as opposed to statistical significance): Statistical significance means the likelihood that the difference found between groups could have occurred by chance alone. In most clinical trials, a result is statistically significant if the difference between groups could have occurred by chance alone in less than 1 time in 20. This is expressed as a $p$ value $< 0.05$. Remember that a trivial difference can have a very low $p$ value if the number of subjects is large enough! Clinical significance has little to do with statistics and is a matter of judgement. It answers the question 'Is the difference between groups large enough to be worth achieving?' Studies can be statistically significant yet clinically insignificant.

**Cochrane Centre**: An institute forming a part of a collaboration who create and maintain systematic reviews of the medical literature. There is no veterinary equivalent.

**Cohort study**: A study in which two groups (cohorts) of animals are identified. One group represents a cohort of animals exposed to a putative cause of an outcome, while the other is a cohort free from this exposure. The cohorts are examined for the outcome of interest in order to test the association of the putative cause with the outcome.

**Co-interventions**: Any intervention (e.g. treatment) given to animals in a study group other than the intervention being studied. Co-interventions in a non-blinded study allow the introduction of considerable bias. The use of additional treatments in an investigation of a particular treatment reduces the power of the study.

**Co-morbidity**: The existence of disease other than the disease of interest in animals that are the subject of a study.

**Comparison group**: A group of animals to which the intervention group is compared. In a trial of a new therapy the ideal comparison groups might be a control group receiving no treatment, and a group receiving an established treatment.

**Condition independence**: Assumes there is no relationship between attributes (e.g. clinical signs) with regard to their occurrence. By making this assumption the frequency of occurrence of two signs within a disease can be computed from the point prevalence frequencies of each sign.

**Confidence interval (CI)**: Studies are performed on a sample of the population, not the whole population, and so confidence intervals give us some idea of how likely the sample mean represents the population mean. Expressed as the sample mean plus and minus a specified amount they are a measure of the precision of the estimate. The 95% CI is the range of values within which we can be 95% sure that the true value lies for the whole population of animals from whom the study animals were selected. Results from a sample population with a wider range of values will have broader CIs than results from a study with a narrower range of values. Increasing the number of results (animals) within a sample population narrows the CIs. The confidence interval quantifies uncertainty and is derived from the sample mean and the standard error. Note that not all error bars shown on graphs of results represent CIs.

**Confounding bias**: Occurs when two factors are closely associated and the effects of one confuses or distorts the effects of the other factor on the outcome. The distorting factor is a confounding variable. Knowledge is the factor measured by scores from an examination paper. An unmeasured factor (and hence a confounding variable) is test-taking ability or examination technique of the candidate.

**Confounding variable** or **Confounder**: A variable which affects the results of a study, was not of interest, and not avoided through the study design.

**Contingency table**: A table in which the outcomes resulting from exposure or intervention are collated. For epidemiological use, these are normally a 2 by 2 table which record the results of exposure to a causal factor, results of a therapeutic intervention, or the results from a diagnostic test.

**Control event rate (CER)**: The proportion of animals in which the outcome of interest (e.g. a disease, an adverse reaction to treatment, etc.) is seen in the control group of animals (i.e. animals not receiving the treatment).

**Control group**: The study animals that did NOT receive the experimental intervention (e.g. therapy). In an ideal study both positive and negative controls are used (e.g. placebo treated, and an existing well-documented treatment of known efficacy).

**Cost–benefit analysis**: Is an analysis performed by converting effects into the same monetary terms as the costs and comparing them.

**Cost–effectiveness analysis**: Mainly used in human health management to convert health gains such as disease prevention into a financial value.

**Cost–utility analysis**: A method of converting effects into animal (or owner) preferences (utilities) and describing it in terms of cost. Used extensively in human medicine (e.g. cost per additional quality-adjusted life-year, QUALY).

**Cox proportional hazard model**: A type of multivariate analysis that is used to identify a combination of factors that best predicts prognosis in the group of individuals. Can also test the effect of individual factors independently. Analysis used when the outcome is the time to an event. The Cox proportional hazard model is used when practical considerations preclude observing survival time in all patients being studied (mainly used in human medicine).

**Critically appraised topic (CATs)**: These are summaries of papers, which are written to answer a specific clinical question. They are written to help practitioners of EBM by sharing the burden of appraising the literature. There are no sources of veterinary CATs but a good collection of medical examples can be found at the CEBM website (www.indigojazz.co.uk/cebm/cats.asp).

**Cross-over study design**: The administration of two or more experimental therapies one after the other to the same group of animals.

**Cross-sectional study** (Prevalence study): Survey of an entire population for the presence or absence of a disease and/or other variable in every member (or a representative sample) and the potential risk factors at a particular point in time or time interval. Exposure and outcome are determined at the same time.

**Decision analysis**: The application of explicit quantitative methods to analyse decisions under conditions of uncertainty.

**Deductive reasoning**: Goes from effect to cause, e.g. if a cow is pale then the cow may have haemolytic anaemia (see Inductive reasoning).

**Determinant**: A factor that produces a change in the health or disease status of an animal.

**Dose–response relationship**: A situation in which the magnitude of the outcome is related to the amount, duration or intensity of exposure. The change in the outcome may be an increase or a decrease.

**Double-blind**: Typically used in randomised controlled trials (RCTs). An experimental method in which both the animals/owners and the investigators do not know and cannot work out which animals are receiving treatment and which placebo.

**Effectiveness**: A measure of the benefit resulting from an intervention for a particular health problem for a group of animals in normal clinical practice (cf. efficacy).

**Efficacy**: A measure of the benefit resulting from an intervention for a particular health problem in ideal (experimental) conditions.

**Event rate**: The proportion of animals in a group in whom an event is observed. Thus, if out of 100 animals, the event is observed in 18, the event rate is 0.18. Control event rate

(CER) and experiemental event rate (EER) are used to refer to this in control and experimental groups of animals, respectively.

**Evidence**: Evidence is something that serves as proof to support or refute an hypothesis. The best evidence (i.e. the evidence with the greatest validity), is provided by studies with a high power to demonstrate a true difference. The value of the proof provided by the evidence may range from weak to strong.

**Evidence-based medicine (EBM)**: The conscientious, explicit and judicious use of current best evidence in making decisions about the care of individual animals. The practice of evidence-based medicine means integrating individual clinical expertise with the best available external clinical evidence from systematic research.

**Explode**: Permits simultaneous searching of both a broad subject and the narrower subjects classed under it (e.g. searching 'Non-steroidal anti-inflammatory agents' will retrieve articles on NSAIDs in general, new NSAIDs not yet assigned a MeSH heading, plus individual drugs such as 'Phenylbutazone' or 'Caprophen' classed as NSAIDs in Medline). Because indexing norms require that the most specific subject heading available be applied, normally an article indexed under the specific heading would not also be indexed under the broader heading; thus, searching only the broad subject would result in lost references, which have been indexed under the more specific heading.

**External validity**: Are the results valid outside the animal population studied? Are results from studies done on one breed valid for another breed?

**Fields**: Labelled divisions of a Medline record; most fields are directly searchable. Medline fields include:

AU = Author
TI = Title of article
SO = Journal title, volume, issue, pages and year of publication
AB = Abstract (present in about 2/3 of Medline references. *Note*: abstracts are reprinted from the original paper; if the original had no abstract, there will be no abstract in Medline)
IN = Institution
SH = List of subject headings under which the article is indexed, including subheadings
UI = Unique Identifier, an accession number applied to each Medline record as it is entered
PT = Publication Type (e.g. review, randomised controlled trial, clinical trial, meta-analysis, practice guideline, etc.)
RN = Chemical Abstracts Registry Number (useful for searching new or obscure drugs or toxic agents)
RW = Registry Number Word (used for searching portions of chemical names, new or obscure drugs).

**Frames**: Contain data, hypotheses, rules, subprograms and pointers to other frames so that complex interrelationships can be represented within a computer program.

**Gold standard**: Accepted reference standard or diagnostic test for a particular illness.

**Hazard (or Hazard rate)**: The probability of an endpoint. Used as a synonym for harm in some publications. In layman's terms, the failure rate.

**Heuristic**: A rule of thumb that simplifies or reduces a problem. Heuristics do not guarantee a correct solution. In some cases it may be an estimate based upon intuition not rules.

**Hierarchical decomposition**: The process whereby a hierarchy makes explicit component parts found at lower levels. For example, pathophysiological syndromes (e.g. congestive heart failure) can be decomposed into component part (e.g. clinical signs of congestive heart failure).

**Incidence rate**: Number of new cases of a disease in a specified period/average population during that period.

**Inductive reasoning**: Goes from cause to effect, e.g. if the cow has haemolytic anaemia the cow may have haemaglobinuria (see Deductive reasoning).

**Inferential statistics**: Determines how likely a given result occurred by chance alone. Since we can rarely study an entire population, we study a sample of the population and by inference apply that result to the entire population. All statistics used in veterinary studies are inferential.

**Information**: Knowledge or facts about a particular subject.

**Internal validity**: Are the results of the study valid for the animal population studied?

**Interobserver variability**: Variability between observers. Do two or more radiologists give the same reading from the same radiograph?

**Intraobserver variability**: Variability by the same observer. Does a radiologist give the same reading of a radiograph when viewed on more than one occasion?

**Kaplan–Meier curve**: Used for estimating probability of surviving a unit of time. Used to develop a survival curve when not all survival times are exactly known.

**Knowledge-based systems**: Contained in some symbolic manner, a store of facts, rules, judgements and experience about the problem area usually provided by a human expert.

**Level of significance**: The probability of incorrectly rejecting the null hypothesis, i.e. saying that there is a difference between two groups when actually there is none. Otherwise known as the probability of Type I error. By convention, the level of significance is often set to a $p$ value of 0.01 or 0.05.

**Likelihood ratios**: The likelihood that a given test result would be expected in an animal with the target disorder compared with the likelihood that the same result would be expected in an animal without that disorder.

**Limit**: Broad restrictions applicable to existing search sets; includes designations such as:

Species
English or other languages
Publication types (e.g. review, randomised controlled trial, clinical trial, meta-analysis, etc.)
Year of publication
Latest update.

**Mapping**: A computer process whereby the search system matches a term entered to the closest subject headings in the database.

**Mean**: The arithmetic average in a set of values. The average.

**Measurement bias**: Being studied can affect the outcome. If owners are asked to record the amount of feed being given to their animals they are likely to measure out quantities more carefully for example. The methodology can also affect outcome.

**Median**: For a set of values arranged in order of magnitude, the median is the middle value for odd numbers of values and the average of the two middle values for an even number of values.

**Medline**: An electronic index to the contents of biomedical and health sciences journals published since 1966. Medline includes a large number of veterinary journals.

**MeSH**: Medical Subject Headings, the thesaurus for Medline; a controlled vocabulary providing consistent terminology for concepts covered by the database.

**Meta-analysis**: A methodically prepared overview of published studies. Meta-analyses typically use statistical analysis to summarise the combined results.

**Mode**: For a set of values, the mode is the value that occurs most often.

**Multivariate analysis**: An analysis where the effects of many variables are considered. Can be used to identify a subset of variables that significantly contribute to the variation in outcome.

**Negative predictive value (NPV)**: The percentage of animals with a negative test that do NOT have the disease.

**Neural networks**: Neural networks are computer-based pattern recognition methods with architectural similarities to the nervous system. Individual variables of the network usually called neurones can receive inhibitory or excitatory inputs from other neurones.

**Normal distribution**: Many biological parameters are normally distributed, such as height and weight. Some, but not all, statistical analyses are designed to work on data that is normally distributed. If the mean, median and mode are roughly equal then a dataset is probably normally distributed.

**Null hypothesis**: The proposal that no difference exists between groups or that there is no association between risk indicator and outcome variables. If the null hypothesis is true then the findings from the study are the result of chance or random factors. The overall purpose of a typical study is to 'reject the null hypothesis'.

**Number needed to harm (NNH)**: The number of animals who would need to be treated to cause one bad outcome (typically an adverse effect of a therapy).

**Number needed to treat (NNT)**: The number of animals who need to be treated to prevent one bad outcome. It is the inverse of the ARR.

**Odds**: A ratio of events to non-events. If the event rate for a disease is 0.1 (10%), its non-event rate is 0.9 and therefore its odds are 1:9, or 0.111. Note that this is not the same expression as the inverse of event rate. It represents the chance of detecting an event in a single individual from the population.

***p* value**: The measured probability of a finding occurring, i.e. rejecting the null hypothesis, by chance alone given that the null hypothesis is actually true. By convention, a $p$ value $< 0.05$ is often considered significant. ('There is less than a 5% probability that the finding [null hypothesis rejected] was due to chance alone.')

**Point prevalence frequency**: Disease sign point prevalence frequencies are the expected sign frequencies if the disease is encountered.

**Population**: Every animal that satisfies the inclusion criteria for the study. It can be a group of animals with a defined characteristic (e.g. neutered male cats), or animals in a defined location (e.g. in the UK). It is the denominator in the calculation of a rate.

**Positive predictive value (PPV)**: The percentage of animals with a positive test result that actually have the disease. (Positive predictive value = true positives/[true positives + false positives].)

**Post-qualification**: Used with existing broad subject heading search statements to focus the search and reduce the number of postings while increasing their relevance. To restrict a subject heading to focus, preface the set number with an asterisk (*) (e.g. if set 1 is Bovine Mastitis and you wish to find only papers where this is a central focus, create a new search statement by entering '*1'). To focus a search by the use of subheadings after the set has been created, enter the set number followed by a forward slash and the two-letter subheading designators desired (e.g. if set 1 is Bovine Mastitis, and you wish to restrict your search to 'prevention and control' and 'transmission', enter '1/pc,tm').

**Post-test odds**: The odds that the animal has the target disorder after the test is carried out.

**Post-test probability**: The proportion of animals with that particular test result who have the target disorder (post-test odds/[1 + post-test odds]). Use of a nomogram avoids the need to perform any arithmetic.

**Power**: The probability of detecting an effect in the treatment vs. control group if a difference actually exists. Must also specify the size of the difference. For example, a paper describing a clinical trial with a new mastitis treatment may contain the following statement: 'The study had a power of 80% to detect a difference of 10 000 cells per ml in milk between the treatment and control groups.' Typical power probabilities are 80% or greater. Power = $1 - \beta$ (see Type II error)

**Pre-test probability**: The probability that the animal has the target disorder before the test is carried out. This is normally the prevalence of disease in the population of animals in which the test is used.

**Prevalence**: The number of animals with a disease, at a given point or period) divided by the population at risk at a particular point or period.

Prevalence = incidence × duration
Point prevalence = at a specific point in time
Period prevalence = during a specific period of time

**Probability**: The likelihood that a particular event will occur or the proportion of animals in which a particular characteristic is present.

**Production rules**: If . . . then rules.

If the animal is male, then it cannot be pregnant (categorical rules)
If the cow has severe milk fever then she will be recumbent (cause to effect rules)
If the cow is hypocalcaemic then the diagnosis is milk fever (effect to cause rules)
If the scouring calves are at grass then consider parasitic gastroenteritis (association rules)

**Pubmed**: An Internet facility that provides access to the Medline database of scientific publications.

**Randomisation**: A process by which animals are selected for a group by random. This should involve a formal randomisation method such as the use of a random number table (strictly speaking this is pseudo-randomisation), a computer program, or selecting identities from a hat. Some investigators confuse the term with arbitrary assignment (e.g. assigning every other case to one of two groups) which can introduce bias.

**Randomised controlled trial (RCT)**: A true experiment, in which the researcher randomly assigns some animals to at least one intervention and other animals to a placebo, or conventional treatment. Animals are followed over time (prospectively). A blinded RCT represents the best form of evidence.

**Recall bias**: The recall of exposures or events may differ in owners of cases and controls. Questions may be asked more times and more intensively in cases compared to controls. Owners of animals with the disease are more likely to carefully consider whether or not an exposure occurred. Can be avoided by the use of a prospective study.

**Referral bias (Centripetal bias)**: Veterinary schools and specialised referral clinics tend not to see the same range of animals presented to general veterinary practices.

**Relative risk increase (RRI)**: The increase in rates of bad outcomes, comparing experimental animals to control animals in a trial. RRI is also used in assessing the effect of risk factors for disease.

**Relative risk or Risk ratio (RR)**: The event rate in the treatment group divided by the event rate in the control group. Also known as risk ratio. RR is used in randomised trials and cohort studies. When the outcome of interest is rare in the population studied then the odds ratio approximates the relative risk.

**Relative risk reduction (RRR)**: The proportional reduction in rates of bad events between the experimental animals and the control animals in a trial, calculated as (EER – CER)/CER and accompanied by a 95% confidence interval (CI).

**Research question**: The best research question should specify a single measurable outcome, as well as all the conditions and important variables. The question contains the population, the intervention or conditions affecting the study population, and the outcomes.

**Sample**: The animals who satisfied the study's inclusion criteria and who actually entered the study, a subset of the population.

**Scope note**: This defines a particular MeSH heading and explains its parameters, provides synonyms covered by the heading, the year that a MeSH heading was adopted by Medline, previous indexing for the MeSH heading, and cross-references to other possibly relevant MeSH headings.

**Selection bias or Sampling bias**: The sample population chosen is not representative of the population at risk (e.g. animals with advanced disease were compared with healthy non-diseased animals).

**Semantic nets**: Use subjects and attributes to represent objects and relationships between them. For example, Milk fever **IS** a metabolic disease. Metabolic disease **IS** an imbalance between input and output. The system could deduce: milk fever IS an imbalance between input and output.

**Semantic networks**: A semantic net consists of nodes linked by arcs. This structure explicitly describes the relationships between nodes. These structures can be used to represent the pathophysiological and anatomical relationships in a disease process.

**Sensitivity**: The probability of the test finding disease among those who have the disease, or the proportion of animals with disease who have a positive test result. Sensitivity = true positives/(true positives + false negatives).

**Sensitivity analysis**: The value(s) of a parameter(s) within a model is (are) varied while the remaining parameter values are kept constant. Changes in the outcome are monitored. This process allows parameters that do, and do not, contribute to the problem solving in modelling.

**SnNout**: This is a mnemonic standing for 'Sensitive test to rule out a disease'. When a diagnostic test or sign has a high sensitivity, a negative result rules out the diagnosis.

**Specificity**: The probability of the test finding NO disease among those who do NOT have the disease, or the proportion of animals free of a disease who have a negative test. Specificity = true negatives/(true negatives + false positives).

**SpPin**: This is a mnemonic standing for 'Specific test to rule in a disease'. When a diagnostic sign or test has a high specificity, a positive result rules in the diagnosis.

**Standard deviation**: A measure of variability. The standard deviation quantifies how much the values vary from each other. A measure of the spread of individual observations around the mean value of the sample. A normally distributed, unskewed curve will have 34% of the cases between the mean and 1 standard deviation above or below the mean; 68% of cases between 1 standard deviation above and 1 below the mean; 95.5% of cases will be within two standard deviations of the mean (see Normal distribution).

**Standard error of the mean (SEM)**: Another measure of variability. The standard error of the mean quantifies how accurately the true population mean is known. It is a measure of the variability of the mean of the sample as an estimate of the true value of the population mean. The larger the sample size, the smaller the standard error of the mean will be. It is used in computing confidence intervals. In a clinical trial, the larger the sample size, the tighter the 95% CI is around the point estimate of the study.

**Subheadings**: These are generic terms to narrow and focus a MeSH subject heading search. One or several headings may be selected at a time, and 'All subheadings' may be selected when searching Medline using Pubmed.

**Survival analysis**: Statistical procedures for estimating survival (prognosis) in a population under study.

**Symbolic reasoning and structures**: A knowledge-based system may contain symbolic structures used to represent knowledge, relationships and reasoning.

**Syntactical systems**: Knowledge-based systems incorporating symbolic reasoning.

**Testing threshold**: The probability of disease above which we test for the disease and below which we do not.

**Textword**: Exact words found in the title and/or abstract fields; useful for searching if no MeSH heading exists for a specific concept. Textword searching requires the use of synonyms and bypasses the mapping feature that allows 'restrict to focus' and subheading selection. Generally, prefer thesaurus searching (i.e. using the subject or MeSH headings).

**Thresholds**: Testing and Treatment (see Treatment threshold and Testing threshold).

**Treatment threshold**: The probability of disease above which we treat for the disease and below which we do not treat.

**Tree**: A term used in databases such as Medline to describe a classified listing of subject headings, showing broader and narrower concepts.

**Truncation**: Means searching for all variations based on a word stem. The truncation symbol on Pubmed is * (e.g. predict* = predict, predicts, prediction, predicting, etc.).

**Type I error**: Mistakenly rejecting the null hypothesis when it is actually true. The maximum probability of making a Type I error that the researcher is willing to accept is called alpha ($\alpha$). Alpha is determined before the study begins. It leads to a false positive conclusion. Studies commonly set alpha to 1 in 20 (= 0.05).

**Type II error**: Mistakenly accepting (not rejecting) the null hypothesis when it is false. The probability of making a Type II error is called beta ($\beta$). Power = $1 - \beta$ (see above). It leads to a false negative conclusion. For trials the probability of a $\beta$ error is usually set at 0.20 or 20% probability (i.e. a 20% chance of missing a true difference).

**Utilities**: Are a subjective measure of the value of an outcome to an owner. The best utility is given a value of 1.0 and the worst utility a value of 0.0. Every other outcome receives an intermediate score reflecting its relative value to the owner when compared to the two extremes.

**Verification bias**: Occurs when animals with negative test results are not evaluated with the gold standard test.

**Volunteer bias**: Owners who volunteer to participate in a trial may treat their animals differently from how non-volunteers do (e.g. volunteers' animals tend to be better looked after).

**Withdrawal bias**: Animals which are withdrawn from studies may differ systematically from those who remain.

# BIBLIOGRAPHY

Badenoch, D. and Heneghan, C. (2002) *Evidence-based Medicine Toolkit.* BMJ Books, London. [This compact and inexpensive book provides the core information to practice literature based evidence-based medicine. Do not expect detailed explanations.]

Blood, D.C. and Brightling, P. (1988) *Veterinary Information Management.* Baillière-Tindall, London. [This book is about the uses and sources of veterinary information.]

Bonnett, B. (1998) Evidence-based medicine: critical evaluation of new and existing therapies. In *Complementary and Alternative Veterinary Medicine: Principles and practice* (eds Schoen, A.M. and Wynn, S.G.). Mosby, London. [This chapter gives a succinct overview of evidence-based veterinary medicine.]

Friedland, D.J, Go, A.S., Davoran, J.B. *et al.* (1998) *Evidence-based Medicine: A framework for clinical practice.* Lange Medical Books/McGraw-Hill, New York. [This book gives detailed accounts of many of the clinical applications of evidence-based medicine. There is a particularly interesting section on treating and testing thresholds.]

Greenhalgh, T. (2001) *How to Read a Paper: The basics of evidence-based medicine.* BMJ Books, London. [This book is very popular in evidence-based medicine as a guide to reading the scientific literature. The content is excellent with clear guidelines.]

Gross, R. (2001) *Decisions and Evidence in Medical Practice.* Mosby, London. [This book provides a very useful structure for transforming clinical information needs into scientific questions. It is a very useful and instructive book.]

Guyatt, G. and Rennie, D. (2002) *Users' Guides to the Medical Literature.* American Medical Association. [This book is based upon the popular Users' Guides series published in the *Journal of the American Medical Association* as series papers. It is a detailed guide on how to appraise the scientific literature.]

Li Wan Po, A. (1998) *Dictionary of Evidence-based Medicine.* Radcliffe Medical Press Ltd, Abingdon, Oxon. [This is a very useful and interesting dictionary providing descriptions and definitions of the terminology used in evidence-based veterinary medicine.]

McGovern, D.P.B., Valori, R.M., Summerskill, W.S.M. and Levi, M. (2001) *Key Topics in Evidence-based Medicine.* BIOS Scientific Publications Ltd, Oxford. [This is an excellent book covering the core skills required to practise evidence-based medicine.]

Miller, R.A. and Geissbuhler, A. (1999) Clinical diagnostic decision support systems: an overview in *Clinical Diagnostic Decision Support Systems* (ed. Berner E.S.). Springer, New York, pp. 3–34. [This chapter provides a succinct review of CDDSs and the diagnostic process.]

Radostits, O.M., Tyler, J.W. and Mayhew, I.G.J. (2000) Making a diagnosis. In *Veterinary Clinical Examination and Diagnosis* (eds Radostits, O.M., Mayhew, I.G.J. and Houston, D.M.). W.B. Saunders, London. [This chapter provides a review of the diagnostic process and a brief description of evidence-based veterinary medicine.]

Polzin, D.J., Land, E., Walter, P. and Klausner, J. (2000) From journal to patient: evidence-based medicine. In *Kirk's Current Veterinary Therapy XIII Small Animal Practice* (ed. Bonagura, J.D.). W.B. Saunders Company, London. [This chapter provides a brief description of evidence-based veterinary medicine.]

Sackett, D.L., Straus, S.E., Richardson, S.W. and Rosenberg, W. (2000) *Evidence-Based Medicine: How to Practice and Teach EBM.* Churchill Livingstone, Edinburgh. [This is a popular and inexpensive book which has been instrumental in popularising evidence-based medicine.]

Smith, R.D. (1995) *Veterinary Clinical Epidemiology,* 2nd edition. Butterworth-Heinemann, London. [This is an excellent book which underpins many of the principal foundations of evidence-based veterinary medicine.]

The *Journal of the American Medical Association Series: Users' Guides to the Medical Literature* is a series of articles published in *JAMA* to assist the medical profession in critically appraising the literature with regard to the strength of evidence provided by a study. Abstracts of these articles can be obtained by using Pubmed (JAMA Users Guides Medical Literature). Electronic versions of the articles in this series may be found at the Canadian Centres for Health Evidence at www.cche.net/principles/content_all.asp

- Users' Guides to the Medical Literature [editorial]. *JAMA* 1993 Nov 3;270(17):2096–7.
- I. How to get started. *JAMA* 1993 Nov 3;270(17):2093–5.
- II. How to use an article about therapy or prevention. A. Are the results of the study valid? *JAMA* 1993 Dec 1;270(21):2598–601.
- II. How to use an article about therapy or prevention. B. What were the results and will they help me in caring for my patients? *JAMA* 1994 Jan 5;271(1):59–63.
- III. How to use an article about a diagnostic test. A. Are the results of the study valid? *JAMA* 1994 Feb 2;271(5):389–91.
- III. How to use an article about a diagnostic test. B. What are the results and will they help me caring for my patients? *JAMA* 1994 Mar 2;271(9):703–7.
- IV. How to use an article about harm. *JAMA* 1994 May 25;271(20):1615–16.
- V. How to use an article about prognosis. *JAMA* 1994 July 20;272(3):234–7.
- VI. How to use an overview. *JAMA* 1994 Nov 2;272(17):1367–71.
- VII. How to use a clinical decision analysis. A. Are the results of the study valid? *JAMA* 1995 Apr 26;273(16):1292–5.
- VII. How to use a clinical decision analysis. B. What are the results and will they help me in caring for my patients? *JAMA* 1995 May 24–31;273(20):1610–13.
- VIII. How to use Clinical Practice Guidelines. A. Are the recommendations valid? *JAMA* 1995 Aug 16;274(7):570–74.
- VIII. How to use Clinical Practice Guidelines: B. What are the recommendations and will they help you in caring for your patients? *JAMA* 1995 Aug 16;274(7):570–74.
- IX. A method for grading health care recommendations. *JAMA* 1995 Dec 13;274(22):1800–4.
- X. How to use an article reporting variations in the outcomes of health services. *JAMA* 1996 Feb 21; 275(7):554–8.
- XI. How to use an article about a clinical utilization review. *JAMA* 1996 May 8;275(18):1435–9.

- XII. How to use articles about health-related quality of life. *JAMA* 1997 Apr 16;277(15):1232–7.
- XIII. How to use an article on economic analysis of clinical practice. A. Are the results of the study valid? Evidence-Based Medicine Working Group. *JAMA* 1997 May 21; 277(19):1552–7.
- XIII. How to use an article on economic analysis of clinical practice. B. What are the results and will they help me in caring for my patients? Evidence-Based Medicine Working Group. *JAMA* 1997 June 11; 277(22):1802–6.
- XIV. How to decide on the applicability of clinical trials to your patient. *JAMA* 1998 Feb 18;279(7):545–9.
- XV. How to use an article about disease probability for differential diagnosis. *JAMA* 1999 Apr 7; 281(13): 1214–19.
- XVI. How to use a treatment recommendation. *JAMA* 1999 May 19;281(19):1836–43.
- XVII. How to use guidelines and recommendations about screening. *JAMA* 1999 June 2;281(21):2029–34.
- XVIII. How to use an article evaluating the clinical impact of a computer-based clinical decision support system. *JAMA* 1999 July 7;282(1):67–74.
- XIX. Applying clinical trial results. A. How to use an article measuring the effect of an intervention on surrogate end points. *JAMA* 1999 Aug 25;282(8):771–8.
- XIX Applying clinical trial results. B. Guidelines for determining whether a drug is exerting (more than) a class effect. *JAMA* 1999 Oct 13;282(14):1371–7.
- XX. Integrating research evidence with the care of the individual patient. *JAMA* 2000 June 7;283(21):2829–36.
- XXI. Using electronic health information resources in evidence-based practice. *JAMA* 2000 Apr 12;283(14):1875–9.
- XXII. How to use articles about clinical decision rules. *JAMA* 2000 July 5;284(1):79–84.
- XXIII. Quality research in health care. A. Are the results of the study valid? *JAMA* 2000 July 19;284(3):357–62.
- XXIII. Qualitative research in health care. B. What are the results and how do they help me care for my patients? *JAMA* 2000 July 26;284(4):478–82.
- XXIV. How to use an article on the clinical manifestations of disease. *JAMA* 2000 Aug 16,284(7):869–75.
- XXV. Evidence-Based Medicine: Principles for applying the users' guides to patient care. *JAMA* 2000 Sept 13;384(10):1290–96.

# ANSWERS TO REVIEW QUESTIONS

**Answers for the questions for Chapter 1**

1. a
2. c
3. b
4. b
5. a

**Answers for the questions for Chapter 2**

1. d
2. a
3. g
4. c
5. d

**Answers for the questions for Chapter 3**

1. b
2. a
3. c
4. e
5. c

**Answers for the questions for Chapter 4**

1. d
2. a
3. d
4. a
5. a

**Answers for the questions for Chapter 5**

1.  c
2.  c
3.  a
4.  c
5.  d
6.  b
7.  a
8.  b
9.  e
10.  c

**Answers for the questions for Chapter 6**

1.  Both c and d report the same odds, and are correct.
2.  a
3.  a
4.  c
5.  b

**Answers for the questions for Chapter 8**

1.  a
2.  d
3.  c
4.  a
5.  c
6.  g
7.  c
8.  e
9.  b
10.  c

**Answers for the questions for Chapter 9**

1.  d
2.  a
3.  b
4.  c
5.  e
6.  d
7.  a
8.  a
9.  b
10.  a

# INDEX

Numbers in *italics* indicate figures; numbers in **bold** indicate tables.